RESET

Your

BODY

THE HANDBOOK TO NATURALLY *Grow Younger* AS YOU AGE

D1512105

By: Terry Givens

www.resetyourbody.com

Publishing services provided by **Archangel Ink**

ISBN: 1942761694
ISBN-13: 978-1-942761-69-3

Dedication

To my father Prather "Pete" Blackmon, in the hope that these pages will help someone else's father live to meet the family their son will finally be blessed with...

I love you Pop

Table of Contents

Why I Wrote This Book

I think that far too many people are suffering needlessly. I want to empower people to make better natural lifestyle decisions that will help them lose the weight they want, have the energy they need, end suffering from chronic illnesses, break through the next level in performance, and ensure them a long, happy, positive, vibrant existence.

I want to help people to not live in fear of the future and to not feel powerless about their health. I want to simplify the confusion and show that it's very simple to be the dynamo of a person that you can be. This I wish for you.

IMPORTANT:

Although this book carries a copyright, you are hereby granted permission to print it, copy it, share it, give it away to anyone else, quote it, do anything you want with it – *except* you cannot sell any part of the book or the whole book, or make money from it in any way, or assist anyone else in making money from it in any way. I feel very strongly that the information in this book should always be available for free to anyone who wants to read it.

PART 1:

WHY RESET YOUR BODY

This Is About You

What was the best that your body ever felt? What was the best that your body ever looked? That's what this book is about. This handbook's purpose is to help you regain that optimal point in your life. My job is to get you as close to that point as possible. I will make you believe that you can. I will provide you with all the tools you need to get there. And I will map the path to get you there.

What Is Health?

Let me start by saying that your body is perfect. It's the most intricate, precise, well-balanced, and powerful machine on the planet. It's designed to constantly grow and build and repair itself. All things remaining equal, your body will strengthen and repair itself as its natural state of being…GO BODY, RIGHT?

When you are healthy, everything in life is better. On the flip side, when you are unhealthy, it doesn't matter how great the rest of your life is, poor health will be a dark cloud over everything you do and every thought you have. Got a ton of money? Great! It sucks to be in pain while you're out spending it. On an awesome vacation? Super! Too bad you can't fully enjoy it because of your illness. Have a wonderful family? Perfect! Wouldn't it be better if you could have the energy and stamina to keep up with the kids and enjoy all of the events together? Health is the basis for everything else in life. Wouldn't your life be better RIGHT NOW if you could get rid of some health issue?

So is health bulging muscles? Is health about how high you can jump or how fast you can run? Is health how pretty you are? That's what I thought years ago. But why is it that world-class athletes are dying of cancer just like everyone else? Why is it that super in shape people can have bad knees and shoulders and skin issues?

I received a wakeup call that having a muscularly defined physique has ZERO reflection on whether you are healthy (on the inside - at the cellular level) AT ALL. Superstar athletes develop cancer every day. They develop heart disease too.

This isn't to say that exercising and working out have no benefit to your health. It's critical but it is just a part of your health. The body is more than just muscles and a heart, the parts that many fitness conscious people solely target. Of course, you must exercise. And more importantly, you have to put the right things into your body so that it can naturally and efficiently become a strong, clean, and in-sync masterpiece, inside and out.

A healthy body doesn't have blotchy skin, acne, body odor, or bad breath. It doesn't have the occasional headache, bad eyesight, or dry hair. A healthy body is a vibrant, energetic, glowing structure. It may or may not have six-pack abs. It may or may not be the fastest running in the group. But a healthy body will never have to fear catching the flu every year or fear having to wear glasses. A healthy body can wake up in the morning without having to prop itself up with coffee.

Now, don't go beating yourself up if you feel you've already failed the healthy person test. That's why you're reading this book. Right? Just because your body isn't healthy NOW, doesn't mean that it can't be when I'm done with you. The important thing is, I want you to reset your standards for what awaits you as a truly healthy person. You don't need to settle. Seemingly minor glitches in our body's functions that we take for granted as "just a part of life" or "just something that comes with age?" BULL CRAP! You. Deserve. Better.

Confusing Health Information

Who thinks that it's SUPER confusing trying to figure out what's healthy and what's not?

- Is eating fat good or bad?
- Is it ok to eat meat? Red meat? Pork? Only fish?

- Is it safe to be in the sun?
- Is milk good or bad?
- Is low-fat yogurt the best? Or Greek yogurt?
- Can I only eat egg whites?
- Is it best to skip a meal or eat a salad instead?
- Are protein shakes good for me?
- Do I need to juice every day to be healthy?
- Is sea salt good for me? What about high blood pressure?
- Is cooking food better for my digestion than eating it raw?
- Is organic food nutritionally better? What if the plant has a thick skin?
- How many calories do I need per day?
- Are all calories the same?
- Should I be worried about gluten and wheat?
- Are diet sodas better or worse than normal sodas?
- Which is better: sugar, honey, stevia, agave nectar?
- What's so wrong with Genetically Modified Organisms (GMOs)?
- Do I need to work out in a gym? How much?
- Don't I get enough water from the foods I eat?
- Is frozen yogurt better than ice cream?
- Are cooking spices healthy?
- What are the best vegetables to eat?
- Is there too much sugar in fruit?
- Does cleansing hurt?
- Should I get a flu shot?
- What's wrong with microwave ovens?
- Is drinking coffee ok?

Rest assured. By the time you finish this book you will understand the answers to all of these questions (and many more). And you will no longer have to rely on current news or scientists to tell you how to be healthy.

Getting Old

Remember being a kid waking up on Christmas morning? You were fired up! Full of energy. Running around the house like a chicken with its head cut off. Limitless energy. Does that just fade away as we get older? I. Say. No. You can choose to believe what you like. You have a choice. Believe that as you get older you're just taking one step closer to the grave and you're doomed to enjoy life less and less. OR that you were NOT put on this Earth to suffer. You know that there are others your age with a similar background that have tons more energy, feel better, and live a healthier, more-fulfilled life. The life that you deserve.

I'm not saying that you are wallowing around barely surviving day-to-day, waiting for the Grim Reaper. You're enjoying beautiful days. You're enjoying time with loved ones and friends. You're enjoying your career and giving back to others. The good news is that you can continue doing those things with a significantly higher standard of living. You can increase your enjoyment with an almost brand-new version of yourself where you feel and look your best. Imagine that. You 2.0! Say it out loud: ___(Your Name)___ 2.0!

Since 1900, life expectancy has been increasing in America. Great! But at what cost? As Americans are aging, more and more are being stricken with various cancers, heart disease, diabetes, and obesity. Fifty percent of Americans (every OTHER person) take prescription drugs. What kind of prolonged life are we looking forward to? Who in the heck would get excited about 80-90 years with that kind of outlook? Not I, said the cat! In my opinion, we are being severely shortchanged. Eighty to ninety years in a drugged out, practically crippled state, depending on others to take care of us. Not able to be as mobile and coherent and energetic as we'd like, and not able to make contributions to society. That's not what I'm planning on.

My goal is NOT to keep you older longer. My goal is to keep you YOUNGER longer.

I believe that a healthy human body can live to about 150 years old. What?! Are you crazy, Terry?!

Does that mean that after 80, I'll be pushed around in a wheelchair, popping a couple dozen pills each day just to keep my body running? Will I be connected to a machine that regulates my organs? No. No. No. I think that a properly healthy and regularly maintained body that is more than 100 years old will be just as good as what we see in a 50- or 60-year-old, healthy, active, vibrant body by today's standards. At 80 years old, my grandmother was still out in the field on her farm in Mississippi, digging holes for fence posts and, in her words, "Climbing up trees, then climbing down and chopping it up for firewood!" (I suspect she may have been a bit overzealous in that description, but you get the point)

I'll give you proof, as you read on, how living to 150 is not only possible but it's inevitable under the right conditions. And as you reach the end of that long life, you will pass away, not in pain and fighting some disease or illness, not requiring surgeries and medical intervention. You will pass in a peaceful, respectable manner. My friend — YOU NEED NOT FEAR OLD AGE.

We only fear it because of the examples that we see around us. The stories of relatives and the sickly. Let me remind you that there are many parts of the world where a large percentage of people consistently live past 100. Think about that. Are these just super humans that have been randomly deemed to live longer, healthier lives? Or...what are those cultures eating, drinking, and doing? What daily lifestyle habits have they adopted over the centuries that have unwittingly led to their ability to cheat Father Time and live closer to their full potential? Why can't you start to work those habits into your life? What if you did?

It's not too late to start!

Maybe you're 20 right now and you went to college and put on the "Freshman 15," and you're wondering how to get that off. Covered here!

Maybe you're 30 and you've just had your first kid (fathers seem to gain sympathy weight during pregnancy too) and you're trying to figure out how to get back to the way you were in your 20s. Covered here!

Maybe you're 40 and you can't play the sports that you used to play. Or you can rest your plate on your belly while you're eating and it doesn't fall off. Maybe you're having medical issues forcing you to take a medley of drugs. And the drugs themselves are causing side effects that are just as bad as the conditions they are treating. Maybe you're having those aches and pains, so you've been thinking to yourself, "I'm just getting old." All those things - covered here!

Maybe you're 50 and you're a lot less mobile than you used to be and you're having health conditions and you're more concerned about life-threatening conditions. Maybe you're worried about cancer "happening" to you. (Cancer doesn't just happen to people). Covered here!

Maybe you're 60, 70, 80 years old...The great thing about your body is that once we tip the scales back in its favor, it will start to Reset itself. We just need to get out of its way long enough for it to work its magic.

This handbook will teach you how to handle all of this and more. It will teach you how to do it and why it works. It's important for you to know the following: No matter where you are right now, YOU CAN GET BETTER!

Your body is designed to do two things: build and repair. Simple.

It just so happens that with most of us, in our current lifestyles, we've been putting a little too much of the wrong things in our bodies so that our body has been spending too much time and far too much energy **repairing** what we are inadvertently doing to it. Now is our chance to fix it all and YOU CAN DO IT!

Do you want to look like you did in high school?

You can do it.

Do you want minimize injuries and play the sports that you used to?

You can do it.

It might not happen in the first month. It might not happen in the first year. It took me three to four years for my body to switch over and tip the scales to the point that I couldn't stop it if I wanted to. But I'll tell you this – as long as you don't give up on me, I won't give up on you!

We can do this together, as a team. I'm here to let you know that if you stick this out and you fight, you will reach your goal. You might luck out and this might come easy for you. One month later – BOOM, you achieve what you want. BRAVO to you. But realistically, it's going to take a lifestyle change over time, six months, one year, two years…each day, week, month, I will show you to track your changes and improvements so that you are aware of your wins along the way. Until one day – BOOM! Once it happens for you, you will KNOW it happened. And it will be worth every second. Worth every sacrifice.

Suspend your disbelief for a while. The best way for you to gain value from this handbook is to have an open mind. Don't try to prove yourself right as you read this. And don't try to prove me wrong as you read. Just put aside your ego and your previous experience for now and try to just understand the information that I'm proposing. First, understand it. After you complete the book, AFTER you've tried some of my suggestions, then you can debate its merits. Do you think that you can do that? If you knew all the answers, I don't think that you'd be reading this book now.

Nothing happens entirely by chance. I believe there is a reason that you are reading this book right now. I'm excited for you to find out that reason. Are you ready? Let's go.

My Story

At the writing of this book, I am 40 years old (40 and a half to be exact). How did I end up writing this handbook? Did I come stumbling down from the mountaintop carrying two stone tablets with the secret wisdoms of the ages? Was it a path that I've been on all of my life? No and no. I'm a simple guy from the Midwest. Ohio. Cincinnati, to be exact. So I can tell you with all honesty I was not raised on a healthy diet, lifestyle, and mentality. No way! Being from the Midwest and spending summers on my grandmother's farm in Mississippi, I was raised with two food groups in mind – meat and potatoes. My rules for cooking, as handed down by my Dad, were, "On every plate have a meat, a starch, and a vegetable" and I loved it! I love our Ohio foods. Cincinnati is known for Skyline Chili™ restaurants and I'd put Larosa's™ pizza against any pizza in America!

Juicing and super healthy eating and detoxing are NOT big things in Ohio. It's not right or wrong, it's just not a part of the prevalent culture.

So my diet, growing up, mostly consisted of heavy meat portions and lots and lots of fast food. Up until I was about 32, I ate fast food two to three times per day. Yeah! Don't judge me! Because to me, Wendy's™ was different than Burger King™ – the square patty vs. the char-grilled patty. And who can say no to McDonald's™ french fries – YUM! I'd have breakfast sandwiches at Jack In the Box™ or a bagel sandwich at Mickey Ds, then grab lunch and or dinner at Taco Bell™ or Domino's™ Pizza.

In hindsight, I was also chronically dehydrated and I didn't even know it. I probably drank one glass of water per day. "What the heck did I actually drink back then?" I wondered in my later years. Some sodas, lots of canned and bottled juices, energy drinks, milk, lots of super-sweetened tea and super-sweetened Kool-Aid™. Purple stuff...Sunny D™...ANYTHING but water. That stuff tasted like wet cotton. YUCK.

With that description, you would think that I would have a pretty major weight problem. Well, I never have been one to get fat and gain a ton of weight. Does that mean I'm lucky? Not in my opinion. We all have a weak spot. We have somewhere in our bodies that our poor lifestyle will damage the most. I'll explain this more later and in much more detail, but none of us are immune to poor eating and lifestyle choices. Some people's weak spot is fat formation. Maybe a big belly. Maybe fat on their butt (big ole booty!) or maybe their weak spot is their skin – terrible acne or other skin problems. Maybe their weak spot is their eyes or their lungs – poor eyesight or asthma. Mine was my joints. So how long do you think it took for my poor lifestyle to finally take its toll on my poor, innocent joints? About fifteen years. Yup. By the time I was in high school, my hips were so bad, I had hip flexors that prevented me from running the sprint track events that I loved. (Carl Lewis was one of my heroes growing up.)

So I switched to indoor volleyball in college, since my hips couldn't handle running. But my ankles (more joint issues) were so weak, I constantly rolled them, which put me on crutches and on the sidelines for most of the season. Crazy, huh? I was the darned captain of the volleyball team, but I'd roll the left ankle and ride the pine until that healed, then I'd literally roll my RIGHT ankle soon after I was healed and be right back on crutches again.

After college, I moved to San Diego, California. Ahhhhh, California, the land of dreams. Also had a major shoulder injury from football/volleyball, resulting in shoulder surgery (if I knew then what I know now, I would never have decided on surgery, by the way). Then let's cap it all off with sharp knee pain in my late 20s, early 30s that prevented me from playing beach volleyball for almost two years. So by 32 years of age, I couldn't squat down on my knees and support my body weight. I immediately had to put a knee on the ground and support my weight somehow because that hurt far too much. Maybe you have issues with your knees when you squat down with your body weight on your knees. Sucks, huh?

Then what happened? Well, I was minding my own business and I attended an Anthony Robbins event. Yes, the renowned and masterful business and life transformation coach himself. It was the Unleash the Power Within event. Four days of powerful insight and business knowledge and breaking through boundaries to reach the next level in your growth towards your personal success. So imagine my annoyance when day four came along and it was all about health…HEALTH?! "Who cares about health?!" I said to myself. "I have muscles, how about I teach health day" were my exact thoughts. That was the furthest thing from my mind at the time. But, good thing for me, I went anyway. (It was a $1,700 event. I wanted to get my money's worth.)

That was the single day that ended up changing my life. Sounds cheesy and cliché, but if an experience or event has ever changed your life, you know exactly what I'm talking about. The teachings of Anthony Robbins that day helped me to grasp the difference between fitness and health. They are two TOTALLY separate things. That day sparked the fire in me that started me devouring health information. Close to 100 books on health and wellness and alternative healing. Hundreds of hours of health documentaries. Hundreds of hours of seminars, workshops, webinars…I even got certified as a nutritionist.

Then I began the process that I now call Resetting my Body. Slow changes at first. That led to more changes and more trial and error and finding patterns and setting up systems and duplicating them. After a couple of years, I would post tips on Facebook. People expressed a lot of interest and suggested I set up a blog. "What the heck is a blog?" Then I set up the blog (www.ResetYourBody.com) and got more serious about posting and creating videos and writing posts, and an idea started to form that I could write a book. I have way too much information to possibly make it coherent enough to follow on different posts.

Seven years of personal experimentation and working with hundreds of willing and open- minded family, friends, clients, followers has resulted in the full and complete culmination of my findings, techniques, and philosophies in these pages.

I can proudly say that the 40-year-old Terry could beat the 25-year-old Terry's ASS!! Really! I'm stronger, faster, sturdier, healthier, more attractive, and more modest. HA! The last two points are a bit subjective.

But seriously, imagine that. What if after a couple of years of dedication and following a simple system you could feel as if you were growing younger even as you are aging? What if you could turn back the hands of time and be able to do things that you had written off as pleasures of the past? I can't claim that I've stopped the clock, but I can guarantee you that I've gained back decades of enjoyable lifestyles that will result in immeasurable happiness for me and those around me. This is the future that I wish for you as well. It is here for you to take it. Let's begin.

"After reflecting on my overall health the last 8mths since I have met Mr. Givens, I realized that I have not taken any over-the-counter or prescribed medication aside from 2-3 allergy pills. For someone who is extremely active and in the mix at all times, I am impressed. No aches or pains, hangovers, or colds have been severe enough to "need" these types of intervention.

Stay natural, stay healthy!"

J.B.

You Have To Believe

The first thing I need you to do is believe. There are two types of people that are reading this book right now:

Type 1: Honestly believes that they can drastically change their lives and their health and believe that others in the world have done it naturally. They will fight and scratch and claw until they find the right system and guidance to get there.

Type 2: And I'm talking to you right now. You don't truly BELIEVE that you can get healthier. You don't really believe that you can reverse the years of damage that your body has endured. Remember that Christmas-morning kid I mentioned earlier? Bouncing off the walls with excitement, energy, and annoyingly bubbly? Each one of us used to be that kid.

Then, gradually, every year we got a little less rambunctious. Every year we kind of forgot what that felt like. We got a little more lethargic. We woke up a little later every day. It got a little harder to wake up in the mornings. We got used to dragging along the entire day, just going from one thing to the next. Over the years, we forgot the vitality and vigor that we had. We forgot what it was like to walk up stairs two or three at a time or run up the stairs! (When was the last time you did that?) We forgot having the urge to jump over a handrail or swing ourselves along a handrail. (When was the last time you did that?)

I'm going to be honest. For me to change your behavior, I'm going to need to brainwash you! That's right. If I can brainwash you to think like me, you'll start to act like me, and then you'll end up with the same results as me. So stop being stubborn and get ready for the brainwashing. Okay? GOOD!

Let's first figure out what beliefs are driving you, which thus drive your actions. Once I can tweak your beliefs a little bit, I'll be able to tweak your actions. Just a little bit every time until one day a couple of years from now, you'll look up and you'll have adopted a TOTALLY different lifestyle, complete with totally different actions. And you'll look at the sky and exclaim "Oh, Terry Givens! You sneaky fox! You got me!"

Why is this belief part important? Because just like anything else in life, if you don't BELIEVE these things that I'm going to teach you will work, then why on Earth would you try any of them? Right?

If you didn't *believe* that a piece of metal weighting 875,000 pounds could fly in the sky, you wouldn't set foot on the airplane would you? If you didn't *believe* that a glass window between you and the 500-pound tiger at the zoo kept you safe, you wouldn't stand there posing for a picture, would you?

If you didn't believe that spending four years in the prime of your life and $100,000+ for a college degree would help you secure a stable, valuable career, you sure as heck wouldn't embark on that journey, would you?

Take a caterpillar. Let's call him Kato. Kato the Caterpillar. If he didn't believe that he could turn into a butterfly, why even waste the time and energy to spin the cocoon? Imagine that this worm-looking thing is making quite the commitment, locking himself into a hard shell on the off chance that a couple of weeks later it will come out as this beautiful, winged angelic spirit. Fortunately, caterpillars don't read the latest scientific studies on the odds of successful metamorphosis. And caterpillars aren't reading Internet articles about caterpillars that failed. And they don't have negative, nay-saying relatives affecting their plan.

If you don't really *believe* that you can turn your health around SIGNIFICANTLY; if you don't really *believe* that you can get off prescription drugs; if you don't really *believe* that you can reduce and remove injuries and illnesses, why would you follow any of my suggestions? It can make all the logical sense in the world to you, but if you don't *believe* that it will make a difference, I guarantee that you won't take the time and the commitment to do any of it. This is where I need to start brainwashing you. (You're getting very, very sleepy...)

We all have beliefs that are very limiting, and those beliefs are causing us to take actions that are preventing us from doing the right thing. The thing that we ultimately WANT to do. But these limiting beliefs don't fit with the health goals that we have. Or these beliefs are causing us to take actions that are ultimately harmful to our health.

For instance, here are my Old Beliefs and the actions that they caused:

BELIEF	ACTION
Many old people have eaten poorly and lived a long life	Kept me eating poorly
If it breaks, there is a pill to fix it	There are no consequences to treating my body poorly

Take your notepad and make a list of your personal limiting health beliefs. Do that now, please. It's important.

Here are some other limiting health beliefs that many have. Ask yourself if you're one of them.

DISEMPOWERING BELIEFS:

- This just happens when you get old.
- It's too much work to be healthy.
- Good food cost too much.
- It runs in my family.
- I need to spend hours in the gym every day to get healthy.
- Being healthy is a lame, boring lifestyle – no fun or pleasure.

Now take a look at your list and really think about what you have written down. Ask yourself:

- Are these quick fixes or long-term thinking?
- Who taught you those things?

- What experiences led to those beliefs?
- Was it marketing from a company that had something to gain?
- Are these beliefs serving me?

Take your notepad and make a list of your personal EMPOWERING health beliefs. What are the beliefs that have helped you throughout your life?

MY EMPOWERING BELIEFS WERE:

- Do little workouts often to avoid having to do HUGE workouts years from now.
- Eat vegetables every day.
- What are your most EMPOWERING beliefs that have helped you? List them in your notepad now please.

Exercise Participation

You HAVE to participate in the few exercises I have in the book. Why?

1. There are no short cuts. For you to really benefit from this, some things are going to be specific to you and your situation, and we need to get that information OUT of your head.
2. You didn't just buy this book to brag about owning it did you? If you're going to take the time to read it, then get serious and try to get the maximum benefit from your time. Your time is valuable. DON'T WASTE IT! So…play along with me.

Get a notepad. This notepad will be used to exclusively track your personal and unique health journey. Yes, you can use a computer file or note feature on your smart phone. You'll end up using it to make lists as instructed by this book. You'll keep a food journal. You'll track your body's progress and changes. You'll set milestones and goals and deadlines in this notepad.

Your Amazing Body!

Millions of people hold as a limiting belief that humans are very frail and fragile little creatures. They think that if some germ gets on them, it's going to take them down. They think that if someone sneezes on them or if they touch a dirty doorknob, that they will be ravaged by the bubonic plague. They feel a victim to these "almighty" invaders trying to destroy their dainty, sensitive body.

Maybe that's you. Are you the one that, every time you see a sanitation gel machine, you dart immediately to it? Squirting it all over? Lathering up? "Gotta protect my weak body from these super germs. I can't get sick! Ugh." Well I'm just making fun (kinda). But think about it. Is that an EMPOWERING belief or a DISEMPOWERING belief? Extremely disempowering! It makes you feel very powerless.

I'm going to remind you that you are in possession of the most intricate, precise, well balanced, and powerful machine on the planet. It's designed to constantly grow and build and repair itself.

Facts About the Human Body:

1. There are 50 billion white cells in your bloodstream whose only interest is to keep your body's natural defenses in good condition (fight bugs, kill bacteria, heal wounds).
2. Each minute, our body is dying. This is a fact. Every 60 seconds our body loses 300,000,000 cells. That amounts to the population of the United States. While this may seem like a lot of dying cells, and you would think our bodies would decay within hours, there are more cells being born every day. Three hundred trillion (300,000,000,000,000) cells are replaced in our body every day.
3. Almost every cell in your body is replaced every three to ten years.
4. We can break our bones but our bones are actually quite strong. One block of bone the size of a matchbox can

support the weight of nine tons, which is actually four times as much weight as concrete can hold.

5. Your kidneys help to get rid of toxins. Without our kidneys, we would die. The reason for this is the amazing filter capacity of kidneys. Each kidney contains one million filters. This means your body has two million individual filters in it that filter out 1.3 liters of blood per minute and expel 1.4 liters of urine per day.

6. Our stomach acids are so strong that they can dissolve zinc. You would think that such a strong acid would eat through our body in seconds, but our stomach lining actually renews itself so fast that there is not enough time for the acid to eat through the lining. If it were not for this renewing capacity, we would have a large hole in our body within minutes.

7. The human body is one big energy-producing machine. When you look at a picture of the human body with infrared technology, all you see is radiating heat. So hot, in fact, that in just 30 minutes, your body can produce enough heat to boil a half-gallon of water.

8. The average person produces enough saliva in their lifetime to fill up two swimming pools.

9. On average, men produce about 10 million new sperm daily. That's enough to repopulate the entire planet in six months.

10. Your immune system remembers all the pathogens that have infected you so that if you catch one of these again, you won't fall ill (the theory behind vaccines).

11. Our eyes can distinguish up to one million color surfaces and take in more information than the largest telescope known to man.

12. Our hearing is so sensitive it can distinguish between hundreds of thousands of different sounds.

13. About 15 million blood cells are destroyed in the human body every second.

14. It is possible for you to survive even after the removal of the spleen, the stomach, one kidney, one lung, 75 percent of the liver, 80 percent of the intestines, and almost every organ from the pelvic and groin area.
15. Your nose is not as sensitive as a dog's, but it can remember 50,000 different scents.
16. Every square inch of skin on the human body has about 32 million bacteria on it, but fortunately, the vast majority of them are harmless.

YOUR BODY

YOU. ARE. NOT. FRAGILE!

We are at the top of the food chain. We eat EVERYTHING else. Remember that!

BUT most of us are in a weakened state right now. Many of us can step off a curb the wrong way and roll our ankle. (I know. I used to do that all the time!) Or have you ever been at work and turned around too fast to grab a file or reached up too far to lift a heavy box, causing you to pull your back or injure yourself? That's a weakened state. It's temporary. You can fix that. Believe it!

Health Challenges Exercise

List in your notepad your biggest health challenges right now. What unique things are preventing you from living a healthier lifestyle? Here are some examples:

Health Challenges:

- Too confused about what's healthy and what isn't.
- Too busy during the day to take time to exercise.
- Travel too much.
- Kids keep you too busy.
- An old injury is preventing more activity.
- Low income is leading to poor food choices etc.

Make your list now please. It's important.

You Maintain Your Other Possessions

What if you owned a $1 million dollar racehorse? Would you feed that horse the cheapest, lowest quality food you had? Even if that food was the most plentiful and convenient? Would you allow your prize horse to loaf around in the barn all week long without taking him out for a workout? Well, we do the same things to our bodies. Your body should be worth $1 million…$100 million…$1 billion dollars to you. It's the only one you have. If you treat yourself with the level of discipline that you treat your possessions, you would show yourself so much more respect.

What about your brand new shiny car? Beautiful, candy-apple red sports car with a perfect wax job and shiny chrome wheels…but going on three years without changing the oil and running on the same three-year-old brakes. You wouldn't dare do that, right? That car is a total WRECK! But you can't tell by looking at it. You can wash the car and shine up the wheels every week, but you never vacuum the inside or clean the dash. That is a very unpleasant car right?

Take Responsibility

We tend to get caught up in the premise that some expert out there knows all the answers that will make our lives better. *The recommended daily dietary requirements by the government are exactly what I need for my particular body to be healthy. The doctors know exactly what drugs I need so that my particular illness gets better.* Have you really thought about that? Six billion people on this planet and each body acts and reacts differently. There is no way a nutrition system or a drug can affect all human beings the same way. We have to start taking responsibility for what we believe and what we do to our bodies. We can't keep waiting for someone to tell us what to do.

For instance, you might absolutely love shrimp. It could be your favorite food in the world, but if you give that to me, I guarantee you, I will begin to wheeze and my breathing would start to become very labored. I'm allergic to shellfish. You have to make decisions based on you and your body, not just the latest fad or the coolest study that just came out. Mostly, you have to use common sense and rely less on experts to tell you how to eat. Listen to your body, my friend.

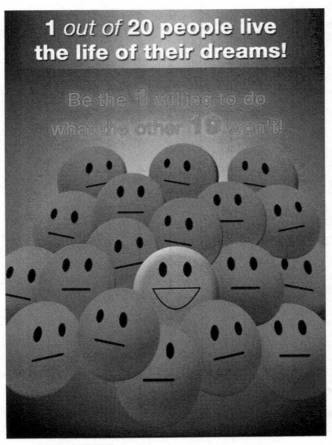

RESET YOUR BODY.com

Statistically speaking, only five percent of people get what they really want out of life. Five percent of people have the career they want; have the family life they want; have the spouse they want; have the freedom they want; drive the car they want; have the health they want; do the things they want.

That's only 1 out of 20 people.

Look around you - which are you?

TIP: If the other 19 people are doing it...DON'T DO IT!

Don't be 1 of the 19.

Basic Health Philosophies

Let's start with a few simple beliefs that are CRITICAL for you to be able to RESET your body. I'll be honest with you. Sometimes belief will be all that you have. At times, it will feel like you are the only one that believes. This is the time when you need to stay strongest. If you are trying to beat an illness or lose fat or have more energy or are worried about someone else, it will be very easy to start listening to the masses and lose belief that you can do it. The tide will turn...it HAS to. Our current health trend is not sustainable. Rest assured, the tide will turn.

Hold onto these five health philosophies...these five health truisms:

1. Your body is created perfect.
2. A healthy body feels and looks optimally healthy.
3. You do not need to slave in a gym to stay healthy.
4. Food is not the enemy.
5. We have 200,000 years of trial and error to find what works and what doesn't.

Your body is created perfect. It is designed to constantly grow and repair itself.

A healthy body feels and looks optimally healthy. No cold, flu, or headache. A healthy body has no body odor and no skin problems, etc. It does not need regular medication.

You do not need to slave in a gym to stay healthy. You do NOT need three hours a day in a gym, seven days a week or a super intense workout and hours of cardio just to maintain your health and fitness. (Working out is important but hours and hours just to KEEP your current weight?…NO)

Food is not the enemy. Real food is great. (Food is a plant or an animal FYI…not the other stuff.)

We have 200,000 years of trial and error to find what works and what doesn't. Seven thousand generations. It's only in the past two or three generations that we've strayed off course.

Believe it. If you really believe in these philosophies, then as you read further you will begin to grasp that this is a super easy problem in our culture to correct, and that we can turn back the hands of time for you to be healthier and younger. Believe it.

Your approach was very appealing to someone with chronic pain, who had exhausted the medical industry's ideas. I've spent literally thousands of dollars on meds. I quit taking them 6 years ago because the side effects were worse than the condition they treated. You know those nasty sick feelings you get when you stir up the toxins? The meds did the same thing. Made me sick consuming them, made me sick getting rid of them. Living the challenges and cleansing is way more pleasant to do, a lot cheaper, and it actually makes things better. Thanks again. Please keep preaching to the masses. To all my friends that read this, go to resetyourbody.com. It's completely free, nothing you have to buy (OK he offers $1 bracelets, but doesn't push them), nothing except a newsletter to sign up for if you want to. Terry explains everything in simple and funny videos and articles.

L.H.

What Is Food?

It definitely IS a daunting and confusing task trying to think of your body as all its separate parts that require specialized knowledge to take care of them. *Ok, I have to eat/do this for my heart, then I have to do/eat this for my brain…oh! I forgot that I need to do/eat this for my muscles.* It would be enough to drive someone insane. Most Americans are well versed on nutrient benefits. At any middle-to-upper class party in America, you will hear conversations about caloric input, protein requirements, carbohydrate fears, and sodium avoidance. But we have been trained to think of food as highly specialized nutrient-delivery machines AND to think of our bodies as specialized nutrient-receiving machines instead of the simple concept that *food is good and your body needs it in its most natural form.* Food! Any food! In any amount!

The question at that point becomes, "What is food?" Such an interesting question for a species that has survived for almost 200,000 years without the slightest bit of knowledge of the amount of calories in a carrot. Or the amount of sugar in watermelon. Or the amount of fat in the meat they ate.

This Is Food:

- Food is a plant or an animal.
- Food is not man made.
- Food has not been overprocessed from its most natural plant or animal form.

The good news is that we have not always had the rampant levels of cancer and diabetes and obesity and other diseases of diet and lifestyle. These are lifestyle diseases from incorrect food consumption. Quite frankly, it's only been the past 50 years or so since the exponential growth of these trends. Fifty years out of 200,000. We can fix this easily. Believe it.

Think of it this way: 200,000 years is about 7,000 generations of families. Think about that. That's 7,000 families passing on knowledge and eating habits from parent to child. Over and over and over. The families that got it wrong developed disease and illnesses and couldn't reproduce to continue to teach the wrong stuff. The ones that got it right passed on those habits and trends to the next generation. This is how traditions and culture are created, through trial and error. Our ancestors figured out what to eat and drink and HOW to eat and drink it or, by definition, they would not have survived this long

It's only been in the last two to three generations that we have been off track. That's it! Simply put, revolutions in technology and industry got us off track. Making food too convenient and thus surrounding us with a wealth of low-nutrient items to eat began the slow, drawn-out process of overeating and undernutrition in developed countries. Lots of stuff to eat to fill our bellies…less and less room in that belly for good ole FOOD.

Nothing is more important than your health. NOTHING.

Please make decisions accordingly.

BE WELL.

What Would a Caveman Do?

When I first became aware and started trying to change my eating habits, I had a simple mental test. "What would a caveman do?" I wanted to be natural and attempt to support the naturally evolved sustainable balance that worked for the first 7,000 or so generations of humans. How would a caveman eat this item? Is this even something that they would have been able to create? The more we muck with our food, the more and more distant it becomes from the natural state that created our coexistence. Would a caveman microwave this? Would a caveman make this protein shake? (Some things require more imagination than others, trying to mentally connect with our caveman brothers)

Let's take a caveman. Let's call him Dave. Would good ole Dave, in his cave, encounter many pancakes? (Batter. Hmmm.)

What about a french fry? - Deep fry a sliced potato in hot oil?

How about a lollipop? – Sorry, Dave. Step one, super-saturating sugar water...huh?

Dave could heat some foods up. He could break plants into smaller pieces. He could mix two, maybe three foods together. That's about the extent of Cave Tech! He wasn't doing a lot of multistep processes to prepare his food for consumption. He just kinda ate it. If it was tough, he chewed it more. If it was hard to eat, he didn't eat it often. If it tasted bland and he was hungry, he ate that too.

You are what you eat right? Literally, your body is as strong or as weak as the building materials used to make it. Low quality foods IN create a weak, damage-prone body. I would argue that a caveman's body was far stronger and more resilient than ours are today. Have you ever been at work and you turned around too fast to grab a file or you reached up too far to lift a heavy box, causing you to pull your back or injure yourself? Isn't that crazy? Think about that. Can you imagine our cave living ancestors whose lives consisted of running on rough terrain and climbing and dodging dangerous animals and falling on the earth?

What if they were so easily injured? (Picture this: Man chases deer. Man rolls ankle on uneven ground. Lion eats limping man. DONE). They were built stronger and they healed faster.

What was the caveman's biggest enemy back then? Heart disease? Diabetes? Cancer? Nope, nope, nope. It was microorganisms. Bacteria and viruses were what kept the caveman down. Infections and non-sanitary conditions lead to short, hard, fast lifestyles for our loincloth-covered pals.

Before you take a bite of that food, before you take a gulp of that drink, ask yourself, "What would a caveman do?"

Simplifying the Body: The Cell Theory

Your body is a very simple mini ecosystem. As long as we keep everything in balance then everything works fine. But when something gets out of whack, your body doesn't just up and die. The other parts of the ecosystem compensate to attempt to keep everything in balance and THAT compensation by the body is what we call disease or illness or injury.

Allow me to explain. (I have to get technical for a minute.)

Your body is made up of a series of organs. Heart, lungs, brain, skin, etc…

Yep…you're basically a skin bag filled with organs – SEXY!

Those organs are made of muscles and ligaments and tissue.

And all of those muscles and bones are made up of cells. **Cells are the basic structure of life.**

Each cell is an individual organism that can eat, move, and reproduce.

Your body is made up of over 100 trillion cells. We are really just a bunch of cells. Cells are super simple. They have one job to do and that is all that they do. You don't have to worry about what body part needs this and what body part needs that, just worry about what a simple single little cell needs. For instance, liver cells have one job: be a liver. Heart cells also have one job: be a heart. Every cell in your body has a single and unique job. So you don't need to be a biophysicist to figure out how to make your heart work better or how to make your muscles stronger or how to improve your liver. The cells already know how to do their job. As the cells get healthier, so does the organ, and so does the body.

We are made of 100 trillion of those cells. But that is not as important as the fact that if you are able to do well by one cell, you can do well by them all. Your entire body's health depends on the health of your cells.

What benefits a single cell benefits the entire body. Believe it.

So what does a cell need?

At a very simplified level, a cell needs:

1. Oxygen (air is not the same as oxygen. Air – the stuff we breathe all day – is a mixture of nitrogen, carbon dioxide, oxygen, etc...)
2. Water
3. A way to dispose of the waste it creates

THAT IS ALL. (Over simplified, but you get the point.)

Think about that for a bit. THAT'S ALL THERE IS.

Let's break that down a little bit more.

Oxygen is the most important source of energy for a cell. Think about it this way – how long can you live without oxygen? A few minutes and you're dead, my friend.

Water is the next most important substance for a cell. How long can you live without water? A little over a week and that's it for you, bud!

Waste removal is critical for a cell as well. The simple act of cells metabolizing creates waste. You don't need to munch down on a bag of Cheetos™ to have waste in your body and cells. You have to remove that waste regularly so the cell doesn't drown in its own garbage.

Nobel Prize winner Dr. Alexis Carrel did an experiment [1912-1940] to keep cells from a chicken heart alive and reproducing new cells for 28 years. Chickens normally live only eight years, so these chicken heart cells far outlived the life of a chicken, and they could have lived on forever if he had wanted. He did this by placing the cells in a saline solution that had the perfect temperature, pH, and nutrient/mineral balance. He replaced this solution daily (cleaning away the toxic [acidic] waste). Eventually, after 28 years, the purpose of the experiment was achieved. The cells did not die of aging. They simply stopped the experiment and Dr. Carrel concluded the following; "The cell is immortal. It is merely the fluid in which it floats which degenerates. Renew this fluid at intervals, give the cells what they require for nutrition and, as far as we know, the pulsation of life may go on forever."

Think about that. Why does the chicken only live eight years when its cells can live 28 years? (Insert "Why did the chicken cross the road joke" here.) Because the chicken is not in its optimal environment. What about the cells in your body? How long can they live in an optimal environment? There are those that say that humans can live up to 150 years in an optimal environment and be happy and healthy and mobile and vibrant at that age. How do you think your cells are doing?

But what happens when the cells aren't receiving proper treatment? They don't just up and die. NO! Cells are not that weak. First, they compensate. Quite often, they will work slower or faster or they will simply mutate. (Hmm, a mutated cell – aka a cancerous cell.) It's just a cell, remember. It has one function and it does it over and over again. Nothing complicated here.

So, in theory, to keep our cells as healthy as possible, we can focus on getting clean oxygen in our bodies, getting clean water in our bodies, and removing waste from our bodies, and we're good to go. That's what a baby has to look forward to. That's all that they have to deal with starting off. If we don't mess it up for them, that's basically all that they need to do and they'll live a nice, long, healthy, happy life.

For the rest of us, it's a bit more complicated. We have spent our lives knowingly and unknowingly not receiving all of the nutrients that our cells need and filling our bodies with toxins and wastes that our cells cannot use, and we have not been removing enough of those toxins and waste. And remember, when a cell doesn't receive proper treatment, it doesn't just die right away

How do we get back on track? It's really simple. But we have to do a little damage control first. We need to focus a bit more intensely (especially getting started) on removing old waste and toxins so that we can equalize our systems and give our bodies a fighting chance to do what they do best – grow and repair. Then we focus on putting clean water and oxygen in (it does take effort to get that oxygen in!) and help our bodies remove waste. That is what this book will guide you through step by step.

What medications are you taking every day?

Goal: 6 Months = cut them in half.

Who wants to get off the meds?

Food Is Not It's Sum Nutrients

Let's take a carrot. Scientist can break down a carrot and analyze what nutrients it has and in what amounts. Vitamins A, B, C, D, calcium, sugar, sodium, iron, cholesterol, fat...on and on. Amazing science! But we can't calculate it all. There are still unknown substances. Any nutritionist will tell you that. So we cannot put all those nutrients back together and make a carrot. As much as we know about food, we really don't know much at all. A nutritionist will tell you that directly. There is some magical, mystical, mysterious thing that we just can't see or measure that somehow comes together to make a living thing as simple as a carrot. Believe it.

That magical, mystical, mysterious stuff? That is what we are missing in a diet based on processed foods. That magical, mystical, mysterious stuff is what science cannot create and put back into food. This is the stuff that our bodies really need to reach their full potential to grow and build and repair.

Just because the label on the box shows that the sodium level is low and the omega oils are high and the protein is high doesn't make that a good, viable food. You know what also has low sodium and high omega levels and high protein? Pond mud! But we know (I hope that we know) that is not food. Food is more than a bunch of fancy nutrients. The more we keep chasing the latest super nutrient, the further we seem to be getting from the health and vibrancy we are seeking. Have you noticed that every two years some new study pops up with a new super nutrient that everyone is chasing or even avoiding? Fat was the enemy for a while. Then protein was great. Then sodium was bad. Then omega oils were the savior. How could cavemen or even animals eat without having access to the Internet and the latest studies to help them choose their foods?

The reality is that when the vast majority of food and beverage choices are processed and separated from their natural state, you

HAVE to know all of the complicated nutrient information so you can try to reconstruct the missing parts.

I'm eating french fries so I have to eat some bran to replace the fiber removed from the potato.

I'm eating canned green beans with a ton of added salt, so I need to drink more water to deal with all the sodium.

Etc...

Or you can consume foods closer to their naturally occurring forms so that you don't need to figure out what nutrients are being removed from your diet.

Rule of thumb: If man made it, don't eat it!

Whole Food Theory

There are those that say we must eat all parts of a food to properly digest and assimilate it. What does that mean? Do we have to eat the skin of an apple to digest the rest of it for instance? Not to that extreme. But your natural body does need food in a natural state (specific proportions and with certain digestive enzymes) to handle food in the most efficient way.

That is what a whole food is: foods that are unprocessed or unrefined before being consumed. That means if it's boxed, bagged, canned, dehydrated, super-heated, has chemicals added, or has a list of ingredients on the label, it's most likely processed. When we remove or add something to a food that obviously changes the contents of the food from its natural state, it's processed.

When we peel a potato and deep fry it, it's no longer whole.

When we put green beans in a can and superheat it (aka pasteurizing – thus killing some of the living nutrients in the food), it's not whole.

When we put meat trimmings and flavorings and preservatives into cellulose then cook it, that becomes a hotdog. It's not whole.

When we shred a sugar cane stalk, crush it to release the sugary juice, heat it to boiling, add chemicals, allow it to evaporate, heat it and turn it into crystals, separate it from the accompanying syrup (that's called raw sugar), THEN send it on to a refinery where it is dissolved, treated with chemicals, filtered, crystallized once more, and allowed to solidify, this time into pure white sugar, you tell me, whole or not?

What about what you ate today – was it whole?

Real food is just as alive as me and you, and the same things that harm us can harm food. There are living enzymes and micronutrients that are alive and have energy. It's that energy that our body takes for fuel. Trust me, you wouldn't have much energy left if you were boiled in water for 20 minutes would you? What if we stuffed you in an oven at 400 degrees for 40 minutes? How healthy would you be afterwards? That's what we do to our live food. The closer a food is to its natural state, the more nutritious it is. Believe it.

In basic simplified terms, your body assimilates and digests food in a specific order and specific proportions and specific amounts. The same order and proportions and amounts that occur in a natural unmodified plant or animal. All plants are like this naturally. All animals are like this naturally. It's nature's little magic trick.

Vitamins and minerals and enzymes, etc., come in and they are then matched up. For instance, you need this vitamin AND that mineral AND this enzyme to fit together, and THEN the body will be able to properly process it and move on to the next. It's like the pieces of a puzzle. Your body is trying to put these uniquely sized and shaped "puzzle pieces" (enzyme "pieces" and mineral "pieces" and vitamin "pieces," etc.) into a completed puzzle so it can then digest and assimilate it. But if for some reason a puzzle piece is missing, then the puzzle is never completed, right? So your body won't digest and assimilate that item. But remember, food, in its natural state, has 100 percent of the needed puzzle pieces, in the perfect order, in the perfect proportions, and in the perfect amounts. Sounds too easy, huh? On the contrary, it took millions and millions of years for nature to harmonize.

This is a very important concept to understand. The further a food is from its natural state the more difficult it is for your body to digest and assimilate it. Believe it.

Surround yourself with people that inspire and motivate you.

Not people that make it ok to just to be OK.

There is no honor in mediocrity, my friends.

BE WELL

How the Body Removes Waste

But wait! So what happens if the puzzle isn't completed? What happens to all of those incomplete puzzles? What happens to the unused puzzle pieces? (Also known as toxins.) Very simple. One of three things will happen:

1. They will be eliminated. Assuming your body's elimination systems are in good working order, and assuming you are drinking plenty of water (soda and energy drinks, etc., don't count remember? They are just another source of missing puzzle pieces) AND assuming your meals don't take days and days to go from your mouth to the porcelain burial ground, your body will quickly and easily eliminate them through the normal channels. No mess, no fuss. Voila.

OR

2. Some of those partial puzzles will be stored for later use. Your body assumes that the missing piece is coming right along. How does it store that for later use? Fat cells. It wraps it up in a fat cell (sometimes to protect you from it). It's not quite a digestible food, but it's pretty darn close. So let's keep it around in case it comes in handy. Or, since we can't get it out of the body, let's wrap it up to keep it contained.

OR

3. Puzzle pieces end up everywhere. Some of those pieces will find their way into the countless nooks and crannies of your body (like breaking open a bag of flour in a room and cranking up a fan). They get into the darndest places! Those pesky little pieces can start to clog up passageways. Or they start to irritate tissue. Or they begin to hamper the operations of the system they landed in. Try pouring sand into a car engine and see what kind of damage it causes.

Common sense. Right? Not a lot of magic here. It's the same logic and experiences that apply to the debris and clutter that we encounter every day. The same is true at a microscopic level. Just because you can't see it, don't assume what's going on inside is any different than what's going on outside. Believe it.

I was a size 18-20 in 2012 and now I'm an 8! I started the Water Challenge in Feb of this year! Weight was 200 lbs in 2012 now I am 150lbs. I was on five to six 20 oz. Mt.Dews a day then!! I did the Water Challenge for 4 months before trying the Salad Challenge and now I am on the No Bread Challenge. I lost 2 inches on my waist doing the Salad Challenge!!

Also I have mild rheumatoid arthritis and moderate Fibromyalgia. So I have to be careful on pushing the fitness. Tai Chi seems to help the best and a little Zumba or dance of some kind. I also try to walk when I can.

During all this, my Fibro and RA have gotten 10 times better and do not flare as often. I am getting to where I can almost live a halfway normal life again and enjoy the things I used to. My goal weight is 120. And healthy.

It works! I love it!

HJ

What Is a Toxin?

So what REALLY is a toxin? Is it a magical, super-evil creation by the government that makes people sick? Is it a set of special chemicals and poisons that are born when humans and animals interact? (I've heard some crazy guesses by people.)

No. A TOXIN is a fancy yet simple name for any substance that the cells of your body don't need as sustenance or that can harm the cell.

Examples:

- Certainly, snake venom is a toxin.
- We are made up of trillions of cells. Those cells produce waste as they perform their bodily functions. That waste is a toxin.
- Carbon dioxide at too high a level is a toxin.
- The preservatives used to keep some packaged food fresh for months or years are toxins.
- Unmatched "puzzle pieces" from non-whole food are toxins.
- Chemicals and medications can be toxins too.

The tricky part is that none of these things cause an immediate effect in the small doses that they normally occur in (except that pesky snake venom) so it's VERY easy to downplay the toxic nature of it.

But what if you were given a pint of any of the above toxins and asked to drink it? That would have a very immediate negative effect. Well, guess what? If you are consuming or using items that keep depositing trace amounts of toxins daily, and you aren't eliminating enough of them regularly, that adds up every day, every day, every day.

SIDE NOTE: Protein powder. How far would you guess that protein powders are from their original natural state? Do you even know by looking at it what protein powder is? Have you ever seen a pack of proteins running in the wild?

No, no, no!

I hate to be the bearer of bad news, but America's addiction to protein supplements is bad news. And let's face it, the majority of people that are adding protein powders to their smoothies and shakes don't even know WHY they are doing it! They heard of other people doing it or it's part of a recipe they found online or some bodybuilder turned them on to it. Do you have a protein deficiency? I can at least understand why body builders use protein supplements (to give their bodies the building blocks to create muscle; when I was a teenager, I used protein powder to gain 30 pounds). What about the other few million people? What do you think you will be missing out on if you don't add protein to your smoothie? Nutrients? Fiber? Live enzymes? More energy?

FIRST OFF: Protein supplements are a solution for 1) vegetarians who want to increase their protein intake or 2) individuals intending to gain weight or muscle mass. Period.

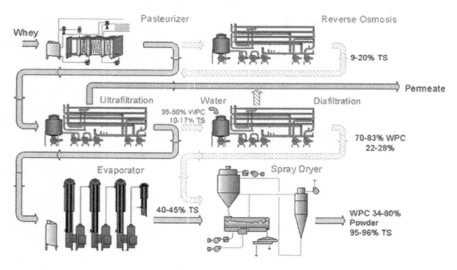

SECOND: It's a powder! Imagine how many puzzle pieces are missing and removed to make this convenient little dust. Pasteurizing, dehydrating, filtering, evaporating, fat isolating. Nature did not intend for protein to be isolated. It denatures the amino acids; it's hard to absorb without dietary fats; and, if they aren't eliminated, the unmatched puzzle pieces build up over time. Do you know anyone that takes a lot of protein powder that is always getting a cold or the flu? Their body is trying to sneeze, cough, sweat, poop, puke those puzzle pieces out.

What about the athletes that have literally been breaking bones in two on live television? Bones protruding through their skin! Athletes tearing muscles in the gym…TEARING MUSCLES?? Those are bulky, beautiful looking muscles built from crap, not quality materials. That is why they don't hold up to the stresses that muscle and bone are meant for. You can't make a tank using plastic parts.

(Healthy protein powder alternatives – gelatin, hard-boiled eggs, raw milk, hemp protein.)

Please stop giving your doctor a job he didn't ask for.

Medical doctors go to medical school to learn how the human body reacts to medications/drugs. They are here to temporarily stabilize us in the case of a traumatic accident or sudden event. They are NOT here to keep us dependent on those temporary measures (drugs, surgery, etc.) for the rest of our lives. They are NOT here to advise you on nutrition and how to eat food. They are NOT here to tell you how to interpret your body's unique response to millions of things that can happen to your body on any given day. Let's stop putting so much pressure on these fine, well-intended servants of our society.

Take responsibility for what happens to YOUR body.

Set a goal to find a natural, more sustainable way to improve your health and wean off of daily drugs and medication.

Research and educate yourself on people that have successfully healed themselves/improved their health without relying on medication permanently.

Are you up to the Challenge?

BE WELL.

Daily Toxic Intake

The great news is that there are many people that have NOT fallen into a toxin-filled food lifestyle. They have eaten clean all their lives. Whole and organic foods. Lots of fresh water. Active lifestyle. They are not putting anything bad into their temple of a body. Why would someone like that need to RESET his or her body? There's nothing bad that needs to be RESET. Right?

Well, the reality is what we consume is only a portion – a rather large portion, but still only a portion – of what ends up inside our bodies.

For argument's sake, let's say that these are the toxic threats that we encounter on a typical day:

Toxins from Air	200,000
Toxins from Water	150,000
Toxins from Food	325,000
Toxins from Beverages	160,000
Toxins from Prescription Drugs	180,000
Toxins from Microbes (Parasites)	525,000
Toxins from Physical & Emotional Stress	200,000
Toxins from Heavy Metals	130,000
Toxins from Radiation (Causes Cell Damage & Death)	230,000
TOTAL TOXINS	**2,100,000**

And let's say, for argument's sake, that the standard healthy body can remove about 1 million toxins in a day. That still leaves over a million toxic elements that accumulate. Then it repeats the next day. And the next. And so on.

Let's look at it this way...

Daily Toxin Intake

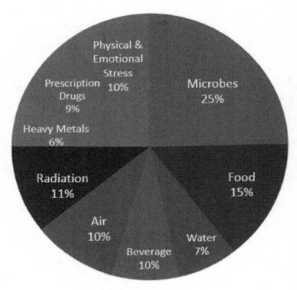

This paints a pretty clear picture of what's going on. This chart helps us see a few interesting things:

1. Things we put into our mouths (water, food, beverages) account for only 30 percent of daily toxic intake.

2. It's also interesting to note that if we were to take out the toxins from food and beverages and drugs and radiation and heavy metals and air (all modern-day toxins), we would clearly see what our ancestors had as their biggest enemy to health: microbes. Bacteria, viruses, parasites. Those have historically been the enemy of man.

What does this tell us? To stay truly healthy and clean, inside and out, we need to do more than just take care to minimize the amount of bad things that we intentionally put in our body. We must also incorporate ways to remove debris that finds its way into us inadvertently from the environment around us. Believe it.

I'll give you a hint: 9 times out of 10, if the media and mainstream medicine are against some sort of food or treatment, I will probably love it and do my BEST to go against the grain.

Why? 'CAUSE THE MAINSTREAM AIN'T WORKIN'! Too much obesity, cancer, heart disease, and diabetes. The majority of the population!...Don't do what "those" people are doing, PLEASE! (salt consumption, eating fat, cancer treatments, cleansing, etc.)

Be open to something different...

BE WELL.

Calorie Counting

While we are on the topic of toxins, let's sidestep quickly and talk about calories and how calorie counting/burning for weight loss will go down in history as one of the biggest mistakes we made. So I am, of course, a Certified Nutritionist, so I preach to you from a professional and standardized platform of knowledge. But here is the way to tell if you're dealing with a seasoned and experienced nutritionist, one that can teach based on their personal dealings with hundreds of clients and not be limited to the textbook, board-certified curriculum. We, as nutritionists, are taught to teach YOU that:

1) "Any weight-loss program is based upon the principle that when the number of calories burned by a person in 24 hours is greater than the number of calories consumed, weight loss takes place in the individual."

The only problem with this statement is that I have literally hundreds of testimonials from people that have lost 5-30 pounds simply by increasing their water consumption, or by ADDING raw salads to their current meals, etc. So calorie intake vs. calorie burning is NOT the definition of losing weight.

2) "A calorie is the quantity of heat required to raise the temperature of 1 gram of water by 1 degree Celsius."

That's cool math and physics and all, but think about it – I mean, REALLY think about it. What does the amount of heat in your body have to do with losing weight? Unless, of course, we believe that a hotter body actually burns and creates a combustible reaction that literally IGNITES fat (and whatever else these hot bodies are flaming away). If that were true, then simply living in a hotter climate (hey Mississippi and Alabama – both in the Top 10 most obese states) would mean that you're burning more calories simply by showing up!

3) "One pound of fat is burnt by burning 3,500 calories through activity. So, to burn one pound of fat would take 11.5 half-hour sessions of moderate cycling per week."

Holy crap! How scary is that? Six hours to burn a pound of fat! If that were true, and a guy keeps his diet the same, AND this guy wants to lose 50 pounds, how long will that cycling take him? I'll tell you how long: 50 weeks of cycling for an hour, six days a week. ALMOST A WHOLE YEAR. To lose 50 pounds! Who in the Sam Hill would not find that intimidating and downright unmotivating?

Here is what you need to remember about calories:

THEY MEAN NOTHING to your health. THEY MEAN NOTHING to your weight loss. How can you possibly compare a calorie from a Twinkie to a calorie from broccoli? Calories are great for scientists, but they just don't fit into your health strategy.

Calorie burning is a side effect of the weight loss, NOT the cause of it. Weight loss comes from the cellular consumption of excess material. As toxins and fat and other waste are consumed, so goes the weight. You poop and sweat and pee out your weight loss. Unfortunately, it does not combust and evaporate with "calorie burning."

My daughter was having difficulty concentrating in school and on her homework when she was younger. At that time, her pediatrician prescribed Ritalin. He immediately thought she was ADD. After a week on this drug and the highs and lows experienced by a 6-year-old, we returned to her pediatrician and demanded, at a minimum, a blood test. Her test revealed her blood sugar was a continual see-saw effect instead of the steady wave it should have been. Along with her doctor's recommendation, we changed her diet to absolutely no white sugar and nothing with PRESERVATIVES. Which frozen foods, particularly fish sticks and frozen dinners were a big part of our diet. Further, her doctor stated that it is highly probable that in her young adult life she would become an insulin-dependent diabetic. With a change in our diet, mainly fresh food nothing canned or frozen, my daughter, who is in her early 30s, has not been on any medications for diabetes or any other meds to help her to concentrate on her school studies. I am of the same mind as you that food, good food, can be a healing mechanism.

Again, thank you for your time and your forum.

F.R.

What's Your Weak Spot?

So we've learned that unmatched "puzzle" pieces that aren't eliminated from your body end up turning into fat and other harmful deposits as they accumulate in your body, right? So why then can two people eat the same diet and one person blows up and gains weight and another person literally shovels food in their face and never seems to gain a pound? What the heck is going on there?

Here's why. Everyone is unique and has his or her own weak spots. These weak spots are where that person's toxins and deposits build up. They don't just go away.

Which one of these is your weak spot?

- Hips?
- Stomach?
- Butt?
- Eyes?
- Hair?
- Skin
- Joints?
- Back?
- Brain?
- Heart/lungs/kidney/liver?

If your weak spot is your hips then it's very easy to spot. Your toxins end up as fat deposits for the world to see. Same with a stomach weak spot or the unwanted butt weak spot. You're not devouring inordinate amounts of food but the toxins that you do take in find their way right smack dab in your derriere and build up day after day after day. But at least you can see the problem.

What about the person that doesn't get fat even though they have an unhealthy lifestyle? They don't get fat since; that's not their weak spot. No, it's far more nefarious. These unfortunate people's toxins build up in places like their eyes (poor eyesight), hair (unhealthy, bad hair), and skin (blemishes). Or my personal weak spot, joints. I was one of those people that ate poorly and never drank water (believe it or not, you can live an entire life on soda and Kool-Aid and juices and other liquids). I never got fat and I ate fast food at LEAST once per day. (Don't judge me.) But meanwhile, "back at the ranch," I developed hip issues in high school, constantly injured and weakened my ankles playing sports, had bad knees, and needed shoulder surgery. You name it. I seemed very fit on the outside but my diet and lifestyle were taking a toll on me – meal by meal, day by day, month by month, year by year.

And the worst of all weak spots are the organs. Heart (heart disease), lungs (asthma), colon (constipation), and how about the brain? Are those unfortunate souls that appear to be in great health really slowly and steadily accumulating toxins that will someday be diagnosed as what we call Alzheimer's?

Makes you think. Right? Can you see how the skinny aren't getting off any better than the obese? My goal here is not to scare you but to enlighten you, because the great news is that it is exceedingly simple to remedy these problems so that you don't become a statistic someday. You can begin TODAY to take action to help your body do what it is designed to do: constantly grow and build and repair itself. You can RESET your body and start the process that will tip the scales back in your favor. Believe it.

Maybe you're not trying to LOSE anything.

Maybe you're trying to GAIN something in your life.

This might resonate with you.

Why People Get Sick

Achoo! Bless you. Cough hack hack. Pardon me. The all too familiar sounds of a cold or flu. Here's a different way to think about it. Colds and flus are actually the body healing itself. Really!

Your body has a few ways to clean toxins out once they get in. Here are your channels of elimination in the order that your body uses them.

Bowel - The bowel (or colon) disposes of toxins as feces

Lungs - The respiratory system helps by the elimination of toxins when you exhale air from your lungs.

Urinary - The kidneys & bladder filter toxins and impurities from the blood and eliminate them through urine.

Liver - The liver has numerous cleansing and purifying functions, including clearing the blood of drugs and other poisonous substances.

Skin - The skin's sweat glands and sweat and tears have a major role in eliminating toxic substances from the body.

The coarsest toxins are meant to exit via the feces. The breath, stool, urine, and sweat are the main vehicles the body has for getting rid of nasty chemicals.

The system burden of daily toxins – pollution in the environment, as well as our food and drink, in addition to the by-products of our metabolism – is normally disposed of through these four prime channels. Each is important and plays a unique role in dispensing a specific kind of waste.

The colon and bladder are what we normally think of when we say "elimination," with the feces being the solid waste and urine carrying that which is water-soluble. The lungs and skin are secondary routes of exit for wastes in solution. A sure sign that the body is having trouble eliminating what it has been able to detoxify is that you have lung and/or skin problems. Of the finer toxins excreted by the body, your lungs get rid of 70 percent, your skin glands get rid of 20 percent, and your kidneys get rid of 6 percent.

Got it? So coughing, sneezing, sweating, vomiting, even diarrhea are actually the ways that your body is using to get "bad stuff" out. Toxins. What you do NOT want to do is take drugs or medications that will slow that process. Sure, it's a pain in the butt to be coughing and sneezing at work or at school. No argument there. But if you can help your body remove those toxins *faster,* you really will be healthier in the end. But what happens if we consistently, time after time, year after year, use drugs to suppress those annoying coughs and sneezes and other *sick* symptoms? Do they just go away? Magically? You bet they don't! They just get buried deeper and deeper into your body's core systems. Deeper and deeper…until one day, they build up and your body knocks you on your butt with a terrible flu. Or it migrates to your weak spot maybe. It's hard to know exactly what will happen of course. Be assured of this – the toxins won't just magically go away. They have to find a way out of your body. Believe it.

You can make a game of it. Literally every time you sneeze or cough, try to think back and isolate what toxin you just introduced into your system – a type of food, a beverage, an odor, particles in the air, etc. Listen to what your body is trying to tell you. Ask yourself, WHY? What is your body trying to get rid of so violently? That may not be the right thing for you…maybe.

It should not come as a huge surprise that "flu season" in the US falls in January – February if we think about it…

- We spend the entire holiday season gorging ourselves with feasts of processed and less-than-natural foods.
- Colder weather forces many Americans into a stagnant lifestyle: less movement and exercise that help with toxin elimination.
- They don't consume enough water to get toxins moving out – cooler weather doesn't prompt us to drink as much water.

- The cooler weather leads to less toxin-removing sweat.
- These toxins build up, leading to germ and viral and bacterial build up.
- Then BOOM! The flu comes to clean your body out from this perfect storm of toxin build up.

Turns out, more times than not, we eat a cold! And we only get the flu if we need to…believe it.

Germ Theory

This section is for all my germ-a-phobe friends. All my friends that rush from one antibacterial gel dispenser to the next – squirting and rubbing and praying to not contract whatever disease was possessed by the previous customer. All those afraid to eat food that touches a table or, heaven forbid, lands on the ground. (What, no ten second rule, anymore?) I am, of course, giving you a hard time…kinda.

So what about germs? They are the cause for all of all our illnesses, right? Louis Pasteur proved and stated this very clearly over a hundred years ago, right? Kinda.

The germ theory states that many diseases are caused by the presence and actions of specific microorganisms within the body, organisms too small to be seen except through a microscope. The presence of these microorganisms will always result in the disease manifesting.

STAY WITH ME HERE – I promise I'm going somewhere with this.

More specificall,y these are Koch's postulates (*postulates* is a fancy word for rules) for determining the cause of a disease:

1. The organism must be present in every case of the disease.
2. The organism must be isolated from a host with the corresponding disease and grown in pure culture.
3. The organism must be isolated from the inoculated animal and identified as being identical to the original organisms isolated from the initial, diseased host.

4. Samples of the organism removed from the pure culture must cause the corresponding disease when inoculated into a healthy, susceptible laboratory animal.

YES – This thinking led to amazing increases in the levels of human disease fighting and infection prevention. Amazingly beneficial changes for the human race.

YES - Specific microorganisms are ALWAYS found when someone has a specific disease. For instance, typhi. S. typhi is present when someone has typhoid fever and variola virus is present when someone has small pox.

So postulate #1, #2, and #3 hold true.

But what about Postulate #4? **Don't give up on this yet guys. I've almost made my point.**

If we take these same disease-causing organisms and introduce them into a healthy person - for the germ theory to be entirely accurate – 100 percent of the people exposed to that microorganism must contract the resulting disease.

Not 80% of those exposed. Not 90%. Not even 99%. But each and every person that is exposed to that microorganism must, by definition of the germ theory, manifest that disease.

But in reality, science and common sense know this is not true. You've seen it hundreds of times: you get sick and many of the people around you get sick too, but not everyone gets sick. It's been proven in laboratories as well. Not everyone that is exposed to a specific microorganism (germ) will contract a disease. In fact, many of these pathogenic germs are found in healthy people. Yes, healthy people have the germ in them but they don't have the disease. Hmm… So really, the microorganisms act more like parasites feeding off the disease rather than being the 100 percent cause.

Tony Robbins explained it this way. 1981. New York City. Seventeen-week garbage strike. Garbage builds up to unprecedented levels. And millions of rats were alongside the garbage. Rats everywhere. Well, the rats must have brought the garbage, right? Of course not! The rats merely fed on the stagnant unmaintained conditions the garbage strike caused. Rats don't produce garbage, but it surely attracts them. Germs can really be said to be similar.

On his deathbed, Pasteur said that the terrain is more important than the germ. This means the germ is not the final determining factor. If the terrain of the person is healthy enough to fight the germ, the germ is nothing. If, on the other hand, the terrain of the person is weak or overtaxed, then the germ will win.

I tell you this to empower you. It's hard to feel like you can make a difference if you believe that your health is ultimately out of your control (i.e., if you believe that all of your hard work and healthy living will go down the drain if someone coughs on you or if you touch the wrong doorknob someday.) Your hard work and disciple with your health is EXACTLY what will keep you from falling victim to every random germ out there. Your strong, healthy body and immune system are not constantly taxed by toxin-filled food and drink. Your body's defenses will not be wasted fighting your darn food. It will be more than capable of handling millions of contacts with germs that you can expect to experience each and every day.

Most times, we'll do more for others than we'll do for ourselves.

Eat better for your spouse.

Set a better lifestyle example for your kids.

Be healthier for your grand kids.

Slim down for the guy next to you on the plane.

Maybe try a Reset Challenge for them.

Smoking and Alcohol

Raise your hand if you've heard of the French Paradox? The French Paradox is the contradiction between scientific theory and real world facts. Those darn French people are doing everything wrong in terms of health: they eat a high-fat diet; they don't jog; they smoke; and they drink alcohol daily. Yet they have half the rate of heart disease and they live longer than us. WHAT GIVES? Are the baguettes magical? Does romance conquer all?

Well, I guess that would be highly baffling if we focused ONLY on what the French consume, without taking into account what they DON'T consume.

Let's say we have two identical twelve-ounce cups. Into Cup A, I pour an ounce of wine. It goes in just fine. I pour an ounce of wine into Cup B and HOLY CRAP it's spilling over the edge and running down the sides right away. What obvious, logical difference is there with those cups? Cup B has more stuff in it already.

Which of the things that we consume affect our bodies the most? The things that we put in the most, by volume, right? Based on the toxin chart above:

- Most: Drink/Fluids
- Next most: Foods
- Next most: Drugs
- Least: Smoking

Intake	French	Americans
Drink/Fluids	Mostly water	Mostly soda
Food	Less processed / less chemicals	Mostly processed / chemical saturated
Drugs	Lower population medication rate	Over half of the population on prescription drugs

At this point, the American "cup" is already so filled with junk that the relatively small amount of toxins from smoking are the proverbial straw that breaks the camel's back. Our bodies are so overtaxed from fighting the huge amounts of processed and chemical-laden foods we eat. Add that to our lack of water intake and the chemical storm in the sodas we consume, along with the side effects of the daily, constant intake of medication and drugs, BOOM! Perfect storm. Those few ounces of nicotine and those few ounces of alcohol each day (as small as they are) flood the body with too much for it to handle and, all of a sudden, they are blamed for everything, since they are the most obvious pure toxins we're taking in.

So to answer the question: Is it ok to smoke a little or enjoy the occasional cocktail? My answer is yes. I don't believe in living a life of deprivation. I don't believe in not having fun. HAVE FUN. In moderation. You are strong! You can't throw pebbles and harm a tank!

Drugs and Medication

Are drugs bad? Are all of the drug companies in a global conspiracy to keep mankind in an addictive drug stupor and rack up unlimited profits while plotting to keep people sick? No. I personally am not a big conspiracy theory guy, and I don't think that every corporation is out to get us. But I do realize that the nature of business and profit do require a company to continue generating profits to stay in business. If people honestly believe that the cure for what ails them is in a pill or a bottle then it's very logical for an industry to be born from that demand. I paid attention in business class. (Supply and demand. The demand is strong).

No one is forcing anybody to pop over-the-counter medication daily. No one is forcibly mandating antibiotics and cocktails of drugs to counteract the effects of other drugs. We ARE being guided by the current medical experts, sure. But in the end, everything that we do is really a choice. We are choosing the only option that we think is available to us. I believe that once people are given another option, common sense and logic will win out and the vast majority will make a different choice. They just need to at least be educated on other options first.

I, by no means, think that drugs or doctors are bad. The breakthroughs in technology and medication in the past 100 years have allowed us as a species to be able to miraculously survive emergency and catastrophic situations that led to senseless death or lifelong debilitation in the past. Prior to antibiotics, pneumonia was a walking death sentence. Infection rates in hospitals prior to our understanding of germs were astronomical. More deaths occurred due to reinfection from unsanitary conditions than because of the person's actual ailment. Believe you, me, if I am injured in a car accident, I want the best surgeon in the country working inside my body to bring me back to health. I want the best painkillers to manage the blinding pain. I want the best antibiotics to prevent infection. But once I'm healed, then it's my job to get back to normal living without the need for drugs and doctors to maintain my health.

The original purpose for drugs and doctors was to help people when they had a traumatic or acute injury or ailment, as a temporary measure to drastically repair something that the body was overwhelmed with. Drugs and doctors were not originally intended as ongoing wellness measures. They come in. They fix. They go away. Somehow, along the way, we got things out of whack. Instead of living the right way and allowing our lifestyle choices to maintain our health and vitality, we slowly began to let our lifestyle slip because we knew we had a cure to what ailed us in a pill or bottle. Instead of living responsibly every day, we live it up and when our body gives us the warning signs that the damage we've been causing has reached the "red zone," we pop some drugs to combat the symptoms. We stop feeling the symptoms but we keep doing the things that caused them in the first place. Not good.

Am I saying don't visit your doctor? No. I'm not saying that. Am I saying to never use drugs? Goodness, no. I'm not saying that, either. I'm suggesting that instead of relying on drugs to keep and maintain health and vitality, allow your lifestyle choices (eating, activities, mentality) to do that and use drugs sparingly and temporarily to correct the more radical attacks against your body's defenses.

Drugs are typically chemically created substances. Man made. So right there we see a major problem with them not being a naturally created thing that you're putting in your body. By definition, it's a toxin and will not be properly assimilated by your body.

Rule of thumb: If Man Made It, Don't Put It In Your Body

Drugs are not designed to cure the root of the problem, they are designed to suppress or eliminate a particular symptom. If you have a cold, the cough suppressant makes you stop coughing and the decongestant prevents mucus from collecting in your lungs and nasal passages. Just what you want, right? BUT that causes two problems: 1) Now, you're no longer coughing to remove the toxins your body is battling. You're not producing mucus, which is supposed to catch the toxins and viruses and bacteria BEFORE they make their way into your lungs; 2) The actual cause of the symptoms, the core problem, is still present and will continue to cause an imbalance in your body.

We can take an aspirin when we have a headache to relieve the pain, but is that really curing the problem? Your body is not experiencing an aspirin shortage, is it? That's not really a solution for the core problem. It's just covering up the body's indicator that something is wrong. The headache is just an indicator of a core problem – maybe you are dehydrated and need more water, maybe it's a stress headache, or you breathed in some vapors that made their way to your brain and caused major irritation. What we *really* need to do is address the core issue or it never really goes away and it will surely reoccur or, even worse, go deeper into our system to a more vital location.

What if you were driving along and the check-oil light came on? What if you pulled over and removed the indicator light bulb from the dashboard? You start the car back up and voila! No more check oil light! Problem fixed, right? This is the exact same thing we do by taking drugs. We are only addressing the body's indicator, not the core of the problem.

Let's say you have spots on your skin so you use a lotion designed to make the spots fade. You've only addressed the warning signs. As far as skin problems go, an unhealthy liver is responsible for a host of them. Be it dry, itchy skin, skin rashes or acne or discolorations, everything has its roots in the liver. Maybe that is really what you need to address.

Remember the puzzle pieces that our body is trying to complete when we ingest something? Can you imagine how many unnaturally proportioned puzzles will accumulate with man-made chemicals and drugs? Weak spot, here we come.

So what if you HAVE to stay on a medication while you are building your body back up to a strong enough state to maintain itself? What if you HAVE to take antibiotics to deal with a short-term infection that got out of control? By all means, do the wise thing and let those drugs give you the temporary boost that you need to achieve to tip the health scales in your favor – and while you are using them, and after you have completed your treatment, do everything that you can to help those substances to exit your body as swiftly and effectively as you can (high water consumption, high live fruit and veggie fiber intake, etc.)

What if you could start repairing and feeding and strengthening those 100 trillion cells in your body and you could start to wean yourself off of your medication? What if you started feeling well enough to forget to take your pills for a couple of days without even noticing? What if you went to the doctor and she said, "Well, my friend, I don't know what you're doing, but we can cut your dose in half!" It's happened to many folks just like you as they began to reset their bodies.

Your body is not so weak that some painkillers and some sleeping medication will poison you to the point of no recovery. Just do the right things. Know what is going on when you take medication. Let your lifestyle be your health maintenance plan, not your medicine cabinet.

Contrary to popular belief, there is no ONE event or ONE decision that you'll make someday that defines your success or will pinpoint your failure. The reality is, there are countless tiny decisions made every month, every week, literally every day, all day long, that compound to your ultimate success or failure. Career, family, health, financial, life...It's all the same. It's NEVER too late to start making those tiny decisions, TODAY. Success isn't defined by what you did last year, but what you're doing right NOW. BE WELL.

Cancer

This one is a bit of a touchy subject and here's why: Millions and millions of us have had a personal battle with cancer. Millions and millions of us have family members, friends, loved ones that have battled cancer. Are battling cancer. Have lost the battle to cancer. This is a very personal issue. Many people have already formed an opinion based on the experts and the medical community that is battling so hard to help with the fight. We have given ourselves completely to the evidence and heartfelt urgings of our trusted advisors. We had to believe so we could muster the courage and strength to make tough decisions and to be there to support our loved ones through their suffering. We had to believe.

My goal here is not to shake that belief or to make any claims of wrongdoing. No. My intention is to present a thought-provoking idea. It neither proves nor disproves what the mainstream thought is. It merely gives food for thought. If you have a strong opinion about the subject, do yourself a favor here – let your opinion go for now. Don't try to compare this information with your information. Just be open to UNDERSTAND this perspective for what it is: another perspective. They say the mind is like a parachute; it works best when it's open.

Remember earlier when I explained what cells need to stay healthy? Oxygen, water, waste removal. But what happens when the cells aren't receiving proper treatment? They don't just up and die. NO! Cells are not that weak. First, they compensate by trying to live with the lack. Quite often, they will work more slowly or quickly or they will simply mutate. (Hmmm, a mutated cell – aka cancerous cell). Make sense?

If that is true, then when we're dealing with cancer, we're really dealing with some undernourished cells. For whatever reason, they aren't getting enough of what a cell needs to survive or they are so surrounded by waste and toxins they can't properly get cleaned up. They just need more of the good stuff and less of the bad. Basic overview.

What if you came out to your front yard and you had a large patch of brown grass ruining your lawn? What's the cure? Cut the patch of brown grass? That doesn't make any sense. What does that brown grass need? Water. You water dead and dying grass, you don't cut it out.

If cancer is really just malnourished/smothering cells, then what is the best way to deal with that? Aggressively clean the body out and get as much nourishment and oxygen into the body as you can. Let that body do what it does best. Build and repair.

If we look at cancer as a disease that we get when we get old, we have no power. If we look at cancer as a random killer, we have no power against it. You bet there are thousands of people that appear to be living a so-called "healthy life" but somehow "magically" get cancer. How is that possible? It's pretty simple now that we understand this possible explanation of what cancer is and how it can manifest. It's just toxic overload. They never cleansed. They never took the time to get the toxins out. If you don't take out the trash, the trash is still there.

It could have come from earlier lifestyle choices. Even if the person is living a healthier lifestyle now, the old damage never disappeared and it just slowly and methodically continued to weaken and weaken until the cell mutation and cancer reached the tipping point. Over-the-counter drugs from the past, poor diet in the past. Who knows?

It could be that this so-called healthy life was not healthy by the standards of what we know a cell really needs. Eating a low-calorie diet is called "healthy" in our culture. Processed foods can certainly be low calorie, but we know the downside of all those puzzle pieces floating around. Diet colas are considered "healthier" in our culture — instead of sugar, they use chemical sweeteners. That's a huge no-no.

It could be that this person ate everything right and drank everything right, so that wasn't their problem. Maybe it wasn't food. How about overexposure to chemicals from lotions or hair care products or jet fuel from overhead planes or cleaning products or antiperspirant?...get it? There are too many sources to trace it back.

Quite frankly, there are a multitude of "could be's." Countless "could be's"! Without being able to shrink down to a microscopic level and take a tour of each and every part of our body, it's hard to know what series of events lead to someone's cancer. But here's what we do know. If you truly BELIEVE in the explanations so far about WHY we need to RESET, you can see a strong push towards regularly cleaning our bodies – not only on the outside but, even more important, on the INSIDE.

A new milestone today. I used to run marathons. In 1997, I had a doctor tell me I wouldn't be able to walk in 10 years. My condition (psoriatic arthritis) is genetic and degenerative. The doctor was wrong, but not by much. I ran three marathons after the diagnosis, the last being in 2002. My arthritis got so bad that I couldn't run anymore. Some days, walking was excruciating. I committed to the challenges last August and have kept them as a lifestyle. Since January, I've done the juice cleanse and the master cleanse twice. With the changes in diet and the cleanses, my joints have improved so much that today I decided to put them to the test. I planned to run one block. I've tried that several times when I've felt good in the time since I quit running, but not in the last year. I had pretty much given up on it. Most times, I didn't get out of my own driveway. This time it felt so good, I ran a mile. I stopped because my muscles were complaining, not my joints! It's been 8 years since I could run, which, by the way, I love to do. Tomorrow, I'll try again. If all goes well, I'll be back to my daily 3.5 miles in a month. You can't believe how happy I am to have sore muscles from running. Master cleanse #3 starts July 7, to be followed by lots of juice. I am going to find out just how much younger and better I can be. Right now I'm 48 going on 32. Thanks, Terry!

L.H.

I thought I already knew what you were going to talk about, and I've seen enough doctors telling me what I should do. Your session was early Sunday morning. I was late; actually, early for the following session. I just wanted a good seat to hear the next session. Instead, I got a new body. Your approach was very appealing to someone with chronic pain who had exhausted the medical industry's ideas. I've spent literally thousands of dollars on meds. I quit taking them 6 years ago because the side effects were worse than the condition they treated. You know that nasty sick feeling you get when you stir up the toxins? The meds did the same thing. Made me sick consuming them, made me sick getting rid of them. Living the challenges and cleansing is way more pleasant to do, a lot cheaper, and it actually makes things better. Thanks again. Please keep preaching to the masses.

L.H.

We can't freak out about everything that we eat and touch and smell and drink. All we can do is stay diligent to minimize what we purposely put in/on us. And then we can have a regular way of getting out the inevitable bad things that do make it into our system.

Get the bad out…Believe it.

It's common sense that just like any other container (our body is a container you know – it's a skin bag filled with organs and water and lots of squishy innards), if you don't clean it out and it doesn't clean itself out very well, then problems are bound to occur. But how do you clean this body container out without breaking it open and taking a broom and dustpan to it?

That is exactly what the next part of this book is about. How to safely, effectively, and thoroughly clean your body – RESET your body. How to do it so that years and years of damage don't take their toll and begin to prematurely wear the body down in the way that we call "aging" – faster than it needs to.

PART 2:

HOW TO RESET YOUR BODY

13 Core Steps to Reset Your Body

1. 10-Day fasting detox
2. Drink 1/2 ounce of water per pound of your weight, daily
3. Eat three salads per day
4. No bread, no pasta.
5. Shoot for a 70% vegetable diet
6. No fast food
7. Sweat for fifteen minutes weekly
8. Work out four times per week
9. No drugs, no medications
10. Find the proper daily herbal supplements for you
11. Cleanse liver twice per year
12. 10-Day fasting detox annually and mid-year veggie cleanse
13. One cheat meal, once per week

The remainder of this book will explain ways to gradually incorporate these 13 steps into your daily lifestyle so that they become HABITS and you don't have to force yourself to do anything. It will be just as natural for you to instinctively gravitate to drinking tons of water and ordering salads and avoiding breads as it is for you to crave sweets and order sandwiches and chug sodas now. You won't even think about. Just let time and habit work in your favor. BE WELL.

PART 3:

THE 8 HEALTH RESET CHALLENGES

Resetting is like...

As I've mentioned before, Resetting your body is very similar to changing the oil in your car.

We can all tell when our car needs an oil change. It's a bit slower when we hit the gas. Automatic transmission cars stick longer in gear and you feel that jerk when it does shift. The car is just kind of...sluggish (sounds familiar?) But THEN! Right after you change that oil, you're firing on all cylinders! The gas pedal is a lot more responsive. It's like a whole new car (remember that) until the oil starts to get dirty again.

Have you ever seen how pretty and golden new oil looks BEFORE it goes in your car? It's almost clear and very sparkly. On the other hand, have you seen the oil that is drained out of the car during an oil change? Yuck! That can't possibly be the same oil that went into the car. It's dark brown or even black. What happened? Did the oil change while it was in the car? It actually did its job: it kept the intricate car parts lubricated and removed any engine debris and machine wear-and-tear corrosion from damaging the engine. It just starts to catch all of the rust and metal pieces and dust and random debris that build up from the normal day-to-day activities of operating a motor vehicle.

Another way of looking at Resetting...it's like changing the lint filter in a clothes dryer.

When that lint filter is dirty, the air in the dryer is not as hot. The clothes take a lot longer to dry. It just doesn't run very efficiently (remember that). But what happens when you clean all of the lint from the filter? The air in the dryer is much hotter and your clothes come out in less time with less energy used (remember that).

Your body is no different. Debris and toxins also build up in your body and if the level of toxic input exceeds the level of toxic output, at some point you would be wise to "change your oil" or "clean your lint filter."

How do we accomplish that? That's what the **8 Health Reset Challenges** are for. Shall we begin?

What are the Reset Challenges?

The Reset Challenges are eight super simple and temporary changes in your eating and drinking habits designed to slowly and effectively demonstrate to you the value of that particular healthy lifestyle and to trick you (ya caught me!) into adopting them into your day-to-day life. I honestly designed these Challenges so that someone like my dad (a 50+ Midwestern man with no background in natural, health-based living, living on the Standard American Diet) could gradually work his way through them and notice SIGNIFICANT changes and improvements in his health in a short amount of time. All this without needing to try any wild, zany, hippie voodoo stuff!

Reset Challenges are NOT the same as cleanses. It just so happens that three of the Challenges are cleanses, but they are NOT the same.

It's simple – start at Reset Challenge #1 and work your way through each subsequent Reset Challenge (at your own pace) and see for yourself what it does for you.

The first Reset Challenges are relatively easy and they progressively push you a little further each time while leaving you with new, healthier, energy-producing habits that will last you a lifetime.

And if you think that there is NO way that you are going to get up to Challenge #5 and do a 1-Day Cleanse, don't worry about that yet. I have a sneaking suspicion that, just like a few hundred people before you, once you lose 5-10 pounds with the Water Challenge, then another 5-10 pounds with the Salad Challenge, then yet ANOTHER 5-10 pounds and you shrink a couple of belt notches from the Bread Challenge, you will think to yourself, "Well, holy crap, if those other Challenges did all of this for me, I can't image how drastically beneficial one of these cleanses will be!" (You are feeling very, very sleepy…)

**The details and specific instructions (and any updates)
are all available online at:**

www.ResetYourBody.com/ResetChallenges

1. **Water Challenge** – This alone will help you lose 5-10 pounds and explode your energy!
2. **21 Salad Challenge** – Expect to lose 5-10 more pounds and your digestion will improve tenfold!
3. **No Bread Week Challenge** – Students shed 5-10 pounds on average and lose inches on their waist…FAST!
4. **10-Day No-Sugar Challenge** – You'll think you're a limitless dynamo of energy!
5. **1-Day Reset** – In 24 hours, you'll undo a week's worth of body damage!
6. **Veggie Cleanse Challenge** – This simple challenge will literally reverse months of aging and your skin will look younger too!
7. **Juice Cleanse Challenge** – Now the magic really starts! Years of damage reversed at the deepest levels of your body!
8. **Master Cleanse Challenge** – The fountain of youth! A cellular level cleanup like no other.

Rules:

- Print out and fill out the attached Reset Challenge Tracking Sheet
- Start with Challenge #1 and progress your way through each Challenge.
- If you've already mastered the first couple of Challenges, you can skip those and start higher up.
- Have fun! Tell some friends and bring them in on your Challenge too!
- Try to start the next Challenge immediately
- Try not to take more than a week or two between Challenges…

It's called a "Challenge" not an "Easy," right?

You do NOT need to burn calories to lose weight. The weight loss could come from gut waste! The weight loss could come from waste from your cells! Without working out AND while consuming MORE calories: Man loses 25lbs in 2 weeks doing Water Challenge; Man loses 45lbs in 45 days doing No Bread Week Challenge; Woman loses 2 inches doing 21 Salad Challenge. Working out accelerates the weight-loss process, but don't be limited by the calorie math!

See more at: www.resetyourbody.com/cleanse-testimonials

I'll make a confession. I didn't go in this exact order when I started Resetting my body seven years ago. (Firstly, there wasn't a bold, dashing young man that had created Reset Challenges already). I actually started with the Master Cleanse. After I did that for ten days (FYI - I advise newbies to start with five days and add one additional day each year you do it), THEN I started adopting the Challenges into my lifestyle, starting with #1.

Do I suggest that you start off with a cleanse of some sort first? If you want faster results – yes. If you are an especially strong-willed, stubborn person that can stick to a tougher commitment right out of the gate – yes. If you are already familiar with lots of these lifestyle commitments – yes.

BUT…if that sounds too scary to you – NO. If you're not yet sold on the benefits of cleansing – NO.

Suggested Reset Challenge Timeline

Water Challenge	10 Days
21 Day Salad Challenge	7-12 Days
No Bread Week	7 Days
No Sugar Challenge	10 Days
1 Day Rest	1 Day
Veggie Cleanse	5 Days
Juice Cleanse	5 Days
Master Cleanse	5 Days

So if you just ran through each Challenge and immediately started the next Challenge the next day you could make it through in 45 days. We call you a RESET Gladiator!

Another variation is to combine the first four Challenges and do them all at the same time (Water Challenge, Salad Challenge, Bread Challenge, and Sugar Challenge). With no break between the later Challenges, you'd make it through in 21 Days. We call you a RESET Demi God!

But for the rest of us normal, non-overachieving HUMANS, I recommend giving yourself a couple of days (at most a week or two weeks) between each Challenge. And I recommend a month between Challenges #5 through #8 (take a break between those cleanses to let your body take advantage of a significantly cleaner you. So it will look more like this:

Water Challenge	10 Days
Break	1-2 Days
21 Day Salad Challenge	7-12 Days
Break	1-2 Days
No Bread Week	7 Days
Break	1-2 Days
No Sugar Challenge	10 Days
Break	7 Days
1 Day Rest	1 Day
Break	30 Days
Veggie Cleanse	5 Days
Break	30 Days
Juice Cleanse	5 Days
Break	30 Days
Master Cleanse	5 Days

Going this pace will get you through the first four Challenges in a little over a month. Then you'll start the cleansing Challenges and do those once a month. You can comfortably work this pace and complete every Challenge five months from now. That's it — five months from now! By that time, you will have adopted each of these major, yet simple lifestyle habits that will have been reshaping, reworking, and repairing your body for 150 days by then. Imagine how much a difference you will be able to see in yourself. Imagine how different you'll feel.

You can remove the included Reset Challenges Tracking Sheet or print one from online:

http://bit.ly/14K5wNM

1. Fill in the dates based on your planned pace.
2. Mark those dates on your calendar or smart phone with alarms
3. Plan your events, travel, and work around them (no excuses!)
4. Buy a flexible tape measure
5. Fill in your starting weight and your starting total inches

Real talk…Many of you are deathly afraid of the scale. Let's talk about that for a moment. Some of you have been purposely avoiding stepping on a scale literally for years. It's fear. And a strong fear at that. I know. Stepping on that scale and looking at your weight – YOUR WEIGHT – makes it all too real. It's easy to live in denial if we don't see the actual number. "Maybe I'm not as heavy as I think."

The number on that scale DOES NOT define you as a person! It does not show how successful or kind or hardworking or ambitious or committed or helpful you are. It merely shows how much you'll **brag** when we're done.

Use the number to get mad. Get mad at those little decisions you made every day without even thinking about them. How those silly little decisions added up over time. GET MAD and make that your enemy. Make each and every pound your total focus in life to melt off. "We're coming after you pounds!! We're coming to get you, weight!!"

You HAVE to track your weight (assuming that you are trying to lose weight). It's important for you to be able to see progress almost at a daily level. That will be the motivation that you need to keep you on track. Every pound. Every inch. Every ache. Every pain. Every bit of energy!

This is not about perfection!

So many people I talk to want, so badly, to make a change in their health, BUT they are hesitant to even start because they are afraid that they will make a mistake along the way – they will cheat, they might not make it all the way through. They think it's an ALL OR NOTHING thing.

IT'S NOT ALL OR NOTHING

YOU DO NOT HAVE TO BE PERFECT

YOU JUST NEED TO START. THE REST WILL WORK ITSELF OUT

You may need to start and stop and restart your Water Challenge three or four times until you make it 10 days. It may take you 21 days (don't do that) to finish the 21 Salad Challenge. You may cheat every day during the No Bread Week Challenge. WHO CARES!? Do you really think that any of those cheats will leave you less healthy than you are right now, without even starting a Challenge?

Don't be so hard on yourself. Don't assume everyone that is living a healthy lifestyle is perfect and that they don't make mistakes.

NEWSFLASH: TERRY GIVENS IS NOT PERFECT!

It took me a full year to stop eating fast food. It took me years to stop eating added sugar. I have a weak spot for Yoplait yogurt. I cheat with potato chips every time I cleanse. I go way over two cheat meals a week sometimes. I don't drink vegetable juice more than once every couple of months. I go wild at Thanksgiving and Christmas and Easter dinners.

Think about something that you're good at: your current career, or a sport, or a talent you have. You were not born doing it as well as you can now, right? It took practice and patience and a LOT of messing up.

Remember when you were first learning how to drive a car? You were nervous as heck! You had your hands at the 10 o'clock and 2 o'clock positions on the steering wheel. You signaled at each turn. 16-year-old you. And now? Steering with your knee while changing the music and applying makeup (not recommended). What happened? A lot of practice and a lot of screwing up. Just focus on getting a little bit better than yesterday.

Your goal: Every day. Just. Get. A . Little. Bit. Better

Eat fewer chemicals, lose more weight!

You're Not In This Alone

You are now part of a family. You are part of the Reset Family. Don't ever think that you are alone in your journey. You will have tons of support along the way.

1. Tell everyone that you know when you are doing a Challenge

    a. That will recruit others to do it with you
    b. They will hold you accountable when you might feel weak

14. Post it on Facebook, Twitter, etc. (Join my Reset Cleanse Support Group on Facebook.

www.ResetYourBody.com/SupportGroup)

    a. On any given day, hundreds of other Resetters are actively taking a Challenge or participating in a cleanse.

Herxheimer Effect (aka Healing Crisis)

This is a great time to prepare you for your body's magic. A healing crisis is defined as the process of your body temporarily experiencing adverse effects due your body's aggressive removal of previously dormant toxins, bacteria, viruses, and general garbage. You can basically relive the symptoms that occurred when you originally contracted the illness or toxin (e.g., you were five-years-old and you got the mumps, then at ten, you took regular doses of antibiotics for a persistent flu bug you had. At twenty, you worked closely with asbestos in a factory for years.)

As you cleanse, your body will release these toxins in reverse order (last in, first out) and you may experience similar symptoms temporarily – coughing and shortness of breath, skin rashes, foul smelling feces – as they are released and you flush them out of your system.

So the point here is, don't quit if you start to experience discomfort or odd side effects. That's good news!

As your body takes the time to attack these old toxic stores and as your body diverts its energy to healing damaged parts, you may experience some, all, or none of the following:

Headaches, soreness, skin rashes, skin eruptions, red eyes, foul breath, joint pain, tingling, minor pain in areas, twitching, nausea, diarrhea, night sweats, fatigue.

"Who the hell wants to feel all that? That doesn't sound like something that I want to do to myself on purpose!" I know, I know. That would suck if it were permanent. But it's not. It's temporary. And the ONLY reason it's happening is because of toxins and garbage that are ALREADY inside you. Already slowing your body down. Already weakening you. Already clogging up your systems. It's clean-up day in your "house." How does house clean-up day normally look? A MESS. Furniture is moved around. Rugs are taken outside. Dust is flying in the air. Mops are in buckets, the rubber gloves are on, and it smells like bleach. It's a mess. For a while. The payoff comes afterwards. A beautiful, clean, fresh smelling home. Your body is the same way.

Remember, your body wrapped fat around toxins to protect you from them. As you cleanse, your body breaks down that fat, and it frees up the toxins again. You can keep walking around with a body literally built from toxins, or you can take some time and flush that stuff out. But if you have a lot of fat, you WILL have lot of toxins released…it is what it is. BE READY.

Just try to see, in your mind's eye, the repairing process that is going on in each of your body parts.

And a special note to women. Your body will be cleansing itself and different parts of the body cleanse differently. Interestingly enough, women have a cleansing process that happens every month already...hint hint. During these Reset Challenges, your body may feel the need to cleanse more. DON'T FREAK OUT. It's cleansing, not dying...NUFF SAID.

You are hesitant to start because you are afraid that you will make a mistake along the way; you will cheat; you might not make it all the way through. You think it's an ALL OR NOTHING thing.

IT'S NOT ALL OR NOTHING

YOU DO NOT HAVE TO BE PERFECT

YOU JUST NEED TO START

THE REST WILL WORK ITSELF OUT

BE WELL...

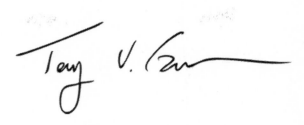

ResetYourBody.com
The 8 Reset Challenges Tracking Sheet
Or visit: www.resetyourbody.com/tracker

Challenge #1 – The Water Challenge (10 days)

Start Date _____	Start Weight _____	*Total Inches _____
End Date _____	End Weight _____	Total Inches _____

Challenge #2 – 21 Salads Challenge (7-10 days)

Start Date _____	Start Weight _____	Total Inches _____
1 2 3 4 5 6 7 8 9 10 11 12 13 14 15 16 17 18 19 20 **21**		
End Date _____	End Weight _____	Total Inches _____

Challenge #3 – No Bread Challenge Week

Start Date _____	Start Weight _____	Total Inches _____
End Date _____	End Weight _____	Total Inches _____

Challenge #4 – 10-Day No Sugar Challenge

Start Date _____	Start Weight _____	Total Inches _____
End Date _____	End Weight _____	Total Inches _____

Challenge #5 – 1-Day Reset

Date____

Challenge #6 – Veggie Cleanse (10 Days)

Start Date _____	Start Weight _____	Total Inches _____
End Date _____	End Weight _____	Total Inches _____

Challenge #7 – Juice Cleanse (5 Days if 1st time)

Start Date _____	Start Weight _____	Total Inches _____
End Date _____	End Weight _____	Total Inches _____

Challenge #8 – Master Cleanse (10 days)

Start Date _____	Start Weight _____	Total Inches _____
End Date _____	End Weight _____	Total Inches _____

*How to measure your Total Inches

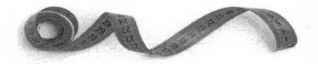

1. Buy a tailor's measuring tape
2. Measure four locations
    a. Both upper arms (mid-bicep)
    b. Waist (horizontal at navel)
    c. Hips (at widest point below waist)
    d. Both legs (mid-thigh)
3. Total those numbers for your total inches

Just finished Challenge #1. I have more energy, my skin is softer, and I lost about 6 pounds. I'm moving on to Challenge #2

S.O.

After being on the Water Challenge for 41 days (no I did not transpose my numbers...haha) I have learned several things.

- Drinking from a small water bottle is not very successful...It is so easy to lose count!

- Drinking from a glass is not very successful...again you lose count, and in my case I really overestimated how much was in it.

- To be successful, you really do have to drink out of a gallon jug!

- If you only drink 1/4 of your jug throughout the day, you don't get much sleep that night when you finish the jug at bedtime!!

- You eliminate drinking a lot of stuff you shouldn't really be drinking!!

- You eat less, because there just isn't any space left in the stomach.

- I do a lot more walking !!...to and from the bathroom!

- I get more time to sit down and meditate...granted it is in the bathroom, but when life is hectic, it is nice to have those extra moments all to yourself.

I am on my 10th day with my jug and I have to admit...we have kind of bonded! I was thinking of making him some clothes to keep him warm on the outside and cold on the inside.

M.H.

I finished the 10th day of the water challenge yesterday. Starting weight 189.8/ Ending weight 189.6 (not as much as I would like to have seen). Starting waist size 39/ Ending size 37.5 (great feeling to lose almost 2 inches on the waist in 10 days!)

A.M.

Water Challenge: I hit my 10 lbs mark…With all the water (WITHOUT Crystal light) and poultry I feel like a water-logged chicken. But I'm not complaining. I'm a 10 lb lighter water logged chicken. Thanks for all the support!"

B.G.

RESET CHALLENGE #1: WATER CHALLENGE!

www.resetyourbody.com/waterchallenge

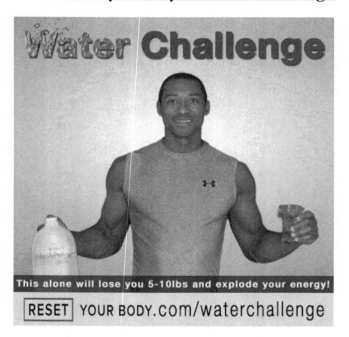

RULES FOR THE WATER CHALLENGE:

1. **1.** Fill up a single jug or bottle or pitcher with your daily amount of water (see below) in the morning. (Buy a jug of water and reuse that jug) You must finish the entire contents of your jug before you go to bed that night. PERIOD.

2. **2.** Do it for 10 days straight.
3. **3.** Finish all of the previous day's water before you start over with today's water. That jug is your lifeline! Only water from the jug counts towards your Challenge. (Squeeze real lemons into the water if you like. Or add sliced cucumbers, etc.)
4. **4.** You can drink additional things. Just minimize the amount of coffee and soda and energy drinks (etc.) during the Challenge. (I don't expect you to just stop cold turkey. I'm realistic!)
5. **5.** Get a group of you to do it together!

Can you last the full 10 days? SHOW ME!

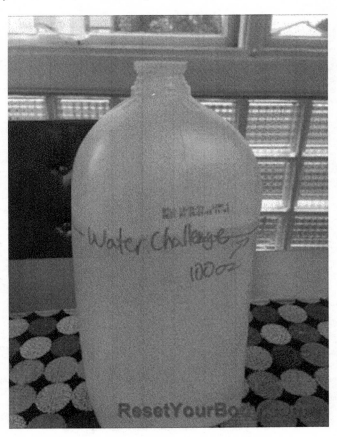

What is the purpose?

Resetting your body is all about undoing years of bad habits and less than perfect health choices. As you've heard a thousand times, drinking lots of water is critical. Quite honestly, the only way the rest of the Reset steps will work is if you keep your water intake nice and high.

What's the big deal about water?

The Earth is 70% water. Your body is 80% water. It stands to reason that water is pretty important stuff, right?

Water is the body's transportation medium. It's how it moves EVERYTHING around to different parts of your body. Water is used to move nutrients to your body's 100 trillion cells. Water is used to move waste and toxins from your cells so it can leave your body. Water is used to wash fat from your body.

These things have to get out somehow, right? They don't just evaporate. So water moves good things around your body, and water moves waste and toxins and fat out.

What's NOT water?

Many of us drink a lot of LIQUID each day but we don't drink a lot of WATER. IMPORTANT – sodas and juice and energy drinks (etc.) are not treated the same as water. Just because it's a liquid does not mean that it's water. You know this already – gasoline is a liquid but drinking it is bad news, right? Look at the ingredients label on a can of soda or an energy drink. That liquid is made of those things: high-fructose corn syrup – is that water? Caramel color – is that water? Phosphoric acid – how about that? If it does not say water (plain H_2O) then your body treats that drink as a food because that's what it is!

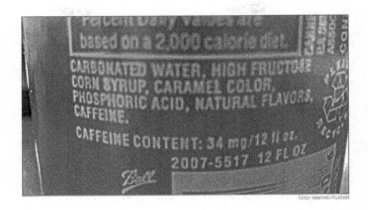

If I take a hamburger, throw it in a blender, blend it up until it's a liquid, that doesn't make it water and your body will use that the exact same way as if you ate the burger. Your body will NOT use it to move nutrients around your body. And your body will NOT use it to wash toxins and fat out of your cells/body.

How much water is enough?

A general rule of thumb to follow is to drink half an ounce for every pound of your weight, every day.

Examples:

150lbs. Half = 75. So 75 oz. each day

250lbs. Half = 125. So 125 oz. each day

(NINJA TIP: For every 64ozs of water, I put 1/2 teaspoon of pink Himalayan sea salt in it. WHY? Increase water intake requires more sea salt to force the water into your cells. – NOT WHITE TABLE SALT! Squeeze 1/2 a lemon in to offset the salt taste. See here for proof - http://www.watercure2.org/mankind.htm)

Things to Expect:

- You will pee more. Welcome the pee! That is how your body removes the toxins and the fat from your cells and your body. Help it out. I drink tons of water and I pee…deal with it! It's temporary – the excess peeing will stop within a week. (Your pee will be very light yellow, almost clear, by the way)

- You'll have more-regular, easier-to-pass bowel movements
- You'll be less hungry
- Many of you will lose an inch or two from your waist.
- Many of you will lose 5-10 lbs. (REALLY!)
- Your skin will become clearer
- You'll have less annoying body sweating (more water = less excess sweat!)
- A few of you will become bloated. That's not because you are drinking too much water. It's caused by a lot of gut activity now that you have the proper amount of water. That's causing some gas, and it's trapped. And, of course, it's temporary.

FACT: When your body has a shortage of water, it takes water from less important places (joints) to use in more important place (brain).

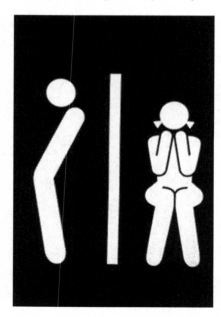

Measuring Results:

- Record before and after weight
- Record before and after total inches

Ways to Make It Better:

- Don't do it alone – get a friend or a group together and keep one another accountable
- Tell others what you're doing – post on Facebook
- Every day will become easier!

LET'S GO!

The goal is for you to adopt this level of water consumption as part of your lifestyle, permanently. If you screw up one day, DON'T beat yourself up. Just finish up what you missed, and start on the new day's amount.

And remember, when you complete this Challenge, start Challenge #2 as soon as you can.

IMPORTANT: Join my Facebook Cleanse Support Group at www.ResetYourBody.com/SupportGroup. That way we can all interact and provide support, feedback, and accountability to one another.

Now, share this with a few people, go fill up your jug, and BE WELL.

Try this! Make yourself a deal: you have to drink three glasses of water BEFORE you can have a cup of coffee.

Took the first two challenges and felt great. I'm pretty sure I lost some weight and inches everywhere! We don't have a scale, I don't measure myself that way, more on how I fit my clothes and feel, so I don't know exactly how much, but was amazing and great. More energy in the end as well. Onto the next challenge.. no sugar. Wish me luck, I'm gonna need it!

S.T.

My wife and I finished the Salad Challenge last night. Really wasn't too bad. We would have a salad for lunch, a salad before dinner, and a salad for snack. Saw some good results this week. Starting waist size 37.5" / ending waist size 36". Starting weight 189.6lbs / ending weight 187.4lbs. My wife dropped 2 lbs and a waist size!

A.M.

I lost 2 inches on my waist doing the Salad Challenge!!

H.J.

RESET CHALLENGE #2: 21 SALAD CHALLENGE!

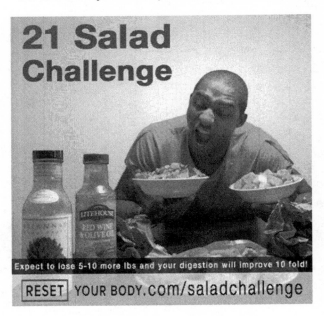

www.resetyourbody.com/saladchallenge

RULES FOR THE 21 SALADS CHALLENGE:

1. Simple. See how quickly you can eat 21 salads.
2. A salad = an uncooked collection of vegetables or fruits (no more than one fruit salad daily). It can be eaten in addition to a normal meal – preferably BEFORE the meal.
3. No more than 10 Days.

Hint: If you eat the recommended three salads daily, this should take you 7 days...Can you do it? SHOW ME!

What's the big deal with salads?

Read on to find out how one salad will change your life!
"Do I just eat salads all day?" – NOPE.

Eat whatever you like. Pizza? Go for it! Hamburger? – NOM NOM! Just add a salad BEFORE whatever meal you eat. GOT IT?

Yep, breakfast too...fruit salad anyone?

Things to expect:

- You'll have more-regular, easier-to-pass bowel movements (nice big ones too)
- Many of you will lose an inch or two from your waist.
- Many of you will lose 5-10 lbs. (REALLY!)
- Your skin will become clearer

Measuring Results:

- Record before and after weight
- Record before and after total inches

What's the purpose?

You are slowly building some core foundational lifestyle habits that build upon one another and create a synergy that helps you remove waste and toxins every day. This is the second of the eight Challenges to Reset your body. When you complete this Challenge, you will start Challenge #3 as soon as you can.

One Salad Will Change Your Life!

Dun dun dun! How's that for a cocky title? "What is this super, wondrous salad," you are thinking? Does it involve super lettuce garnished with chopped unicorn horn from the future? Not exactly.

Let me ask you this:

Do you want one tip that, just by itself, would enable you to eat MORE than you eat now and still lose weight AND have more energy AND improve your digestion? Read on.

Have you heard that iceberg lettuce is pretty much a useless, nutrient-lacking freeloader in the vegetable kingdom that does precious little for your body? I'm going to prove that wrong.

Do you laugh when you see someone eat a salad then slide that bowl aside to devour half of a pizza and end it with an ice cream dessert? I'll show you that that is not the waste of time you think it is.

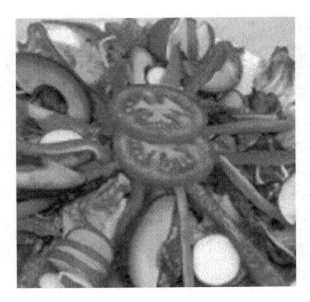

Is your pantry filled with canned food and boxes of food, but no fruit fly-attracting "real" food lying about? I've got something for that too.

Reset Beginnings

When I began this whole concept of Resetting my body five or six years ago, I did three simple things that first year that made ALL of the difference for me:

1. Started drink 1/2 ounce of plain water for every pound of my weight daily (almost a gallon for me)

2. Stopped eating fast food (I used to eat it twice a day…everyday! Yes, me. Don't judge!)
3. Started eating a salad before each and every meal

Number three is what I'm going to dissect today. One thing you'll hear me talk about a lot is eating a salad before every meal. Here in my video on weight loss: http://youtu.be/BhKD3-ty2yU.

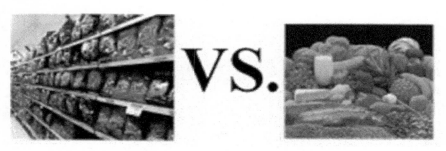

Think about what you've eaten in the past 24 hours. Each and every thing: breakfast, lunch, dinner. All snacks in between. If you eat the S.A.D. (Standard American Diet), this is approximately what you had:

Breakfast:

Pancakes/waffles/bagel

Dinner:

Meat dish
Pasta/starchy dish
Cooked vegetable

Lunch:

Sandwich (hamburger, chicken sandwich, etc.)
French Fries

Snacks:

Candy
Chocolate
Potato chips

Of course, there are many of you out there saying, "Oh, I don't eat like that. I have some fruit and veggies," or "I skipped a meal. I don't eat that much." A) Stop talking to yourself. B) I am sure many of you don't eat this exact menu daily or ever, but the majority of the 300 million Americans do. So for simplicity's sake...humor me.

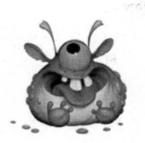

Look at that list again, please. Very few if any of those items have enough live enzymes to help the body digest them. And they certainly don't have enough fiber to help your body smoothly and quickly move it through your digestive system. Do you notice how your belly pokes out after these meals? Why is that? Well, you crammed a lot of dry dead food into your elastic stomach and intestines. They swell up (kind of like when a snake swallows its food whole – YUM!) to fit the food you've eaten. The tricky part is that your stomach doesn't have infinite digestive enzymes and fiber to handle all this stuff we're eating. With all the things in that list being processed (highly altered and modified from their natural state) and being cooked (heating up live stuff tends to kill it – how long would you last if I heated you up to 160 degrees?) the foods in the list above take FOREVER to break down and take FOREVER to travel the 30 feet from your mouth through your intestines and into the porcelain graveyard.

How It Works

With a healthy, properly functioning body (say, that of a child) it should take food about 24-36 hours to make the "round" trip. By that time, your body will have gleaned all of the usable energy and nutrients, and you should expel the same weight of food that you took in...100% same weight. Ate a quarter-pound burger? You'd better be laying quarter pound "eggs" when you're done (don't go for a visual on that, please). That's how a healthy, properly functioning body works.

So what happens if your body isn't working like that? What if you're having three meals a day but you're not having three bowel movements each day too? What if it's taking far longer than 24-36 hours for food to do the Tour De Bowels? What happens if all of that food never makes its way all the way out? NOTHING GOOD!

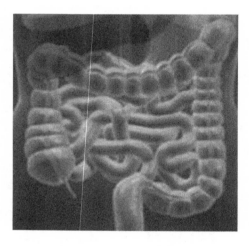

Skip this paragraph if you don't like squishy, smelly things. Your body is a 98-degree container, right? Let's be real here. It's just like any other container, like your refrigerator. Let's fill your fridge up then unplug it during a heat wave for a day or two and then open the door. Funk city, right? Body odor, bad breath, gas, heartburn, low energy, infection, contamination, and malnourishment. You know what's going on in there. It's common sense, right? Now, you're not going to burst and explode into little pieces from the wild chemistry experiment going on in your innards, so you're not going to die overnight or anything. But it sure does put a big damper on a fun, energetic, clean lifestyle?

Happy Ending

GOOD NEWS: Your life is not over and we don't need to bury you. We can take action today, RIGHT NOW, even, to reverse this process and make all the difference in the world...TODAY! We don't need special drugs or chemical laxatives or medication to fix this.

Problem = Not enough live enzymes; Not enough live natural fiber.

Solution = Add more live natural enzymes to diet; Add more live natural fiber to diet. Voila!

(You, of course, will need lots of water and have to rid yourself of bulking breads, pastas, etc. but this isn't about that. This is about salad only)

The solution is to put enough live food IN to balance and digest and move along the parade of donuts and buns and pizza that we can't seem to say no to. (I love that stuff too, you know – and I eat it.)

Your job is to come up with an easy system that you can follow that will realistically help you tip the scale of live food a little bit. One salad before each and every meal. Get those enzymes and that fiber in there 2-3 times per day. You can still eat your meal but eat the salad PRIOR to the meal so that you get your responsibility out of the way first and foremost...then eat up!

What is a salad?

A salad is any uncooked collection of vegetables or fruits. Uncooked is key. We need those live enzymes, remember? Don't go killing off our little buddies. You can make your own salads at home. All you need is lettuce or spinach (I prefer Romaine lettuce) and any type of veggies you like. My favorites are tomato, cucumber, red onions, and carrots. Now add a little sea salt. You can make a week's worth and bring it with you every day to work. You can order a side salad to come before your meal when you eat out. You can have a fruit salad before your breakfast (or just eat an apple and avocado and watermelon slice – same result, right?)

Pick up pre-made salads from the grocery store. Grab a salad at a fast food place. Salads are around us everywhere. Just open your eyes; you will see them.

When the waiter asks what you want, you place your order, and then you add, "Can I start with a side salad, please?" Snack on baby carrots and grapes and easy, convenient live foods. Give your body something to work with.

Salad Dressing

Rule of thumb: creamy is bad (cream comes from milk and who knows how much processing it took). So no Ranch, Thousand Island, anything with the word "creamy" in it. Stick to vinaigrettes (meaning its base is vinegar), Italian, etc.

Here is what you'll notice

- If you're really backed up, you will have gas in the beginning. Why? Do salads give people gas? NO. What's happening is that the live enzymes are doing their job. It's like pouring Drano down a clogged sink (juicing vegetables REALLY accelerates this process). They start to digest and dissolve old food and gas gets released in the process. That darn old food shouldn't be in there in the first place. Burn it out. You don't need it.
- You will have more frequent and regular bowel movements (I talk about that a bunch, huh?) Your goal is two to three times a day, remember? What goes in, must come out.
- You will eat less of the main meal.
- Your belly will get flatter (those three BMs a day are coming from somewhere, right?)
- You will smell better and need to use less chewing gum (all that gas and funk have an alternate route out now).

Why not just try it out for a week? Eventually this will be such a regular part of your lifestyle that you won't ever remember NOT eating a salad with each meal. Just like you are so used to snacking on what you snack on now. You subconsciously do it and don't even notice half the time. This will be like that too. But you have to start and stick to it for the pattern to kick in.

So don't forget your line: Waiter: "What can I get for you?" You: "blah blah blah. And can I start with a side salad please?"

BE WELL.

Blood pressure medication, cholesterol medication, antibiotics, antacids, thyroid medications, etc... Would you like to wean yourself off your daily medications? What if you could cut your dose in half in a few months? (All doctor approved.) Imagine that...

"I went from 13 pills a day, to 1!"

P.H.

"I cut the doses on both my BP medications in half!"

P.B.

How can the 21 Salad Challenge help you eat MORE food and have better digestion, less constipation, and make your skin look 10 years younger? FACT: Billions of uncooked, live enzymes in veggies and fruits LITERALLY eat away at old junk food in your gut to get that old food out of YOU!
Did you know that?

"No bread for one week… Can already see definition changes! I eat a very clean and healthy diet, with exercise/weights 6 days a week! Have been drinking a gallon of water a day!! My energy is awesome…. Can't wait for more healthy results!"

B.N. [Athlete]

The thing that made it click was I could not bend over in my chair and tie my shoes without cutting off my air supply. Something had to happen.

45 days he cut out all the "whites": white bread, potatoes, white rice.

LOST a total of 47 lbs

LOST 6" on his waist

LOST 10" on his belly

LOST 1.5" on his neck

C.P.

RESET CHALLENGE #3: NO BREAD WEEK CHALLENGE!

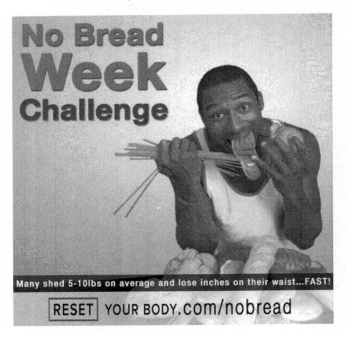

www.resetyourbody.com/nobread/

That's right. NO BREAD FOR A WEEK!

"But why, Terry? Why would you deprive us so?? Have we wronged you??" HA! No, people. Calm down. I will explain. And you will see.

NOTE: This is not about gluten or wheat. I'm focusing on fluffy, clogging processed foods.

NO BREAD WEEK RULES:

1. No foods from the list below for ten days straight!
2. Water, Water, Water – Drink 1/2 an ounce of water for every pound of your body weight daily. Example: 150lb person. 1/2 of 150 = 75. That's 75 ounces. (Soda and energy drinks and juice and coffee DO NOT count)
3. Bring some friends into the Challenge with you!

DO NOT EAT THESE:

- Bread (white, wheat, whole grain, pitas, and any other type)
- Bagels
- Pasta
- Pizza
- White rice, rice noodles, rice cakes
- Cake (cupcakes, Twinkies, cookies, etc.)
- Pancakes, waffles
- Pasta
- Cereal, crackers, chips or any other packaged food
- Granola
- Potatoes (white, red, french fries, potato chips, etc.)

YOU ARE ALLOWED TO EAT THESE:

* Tortillas (corn, flour)
* Brown Rice (not every day)
* Oatmeal (not every day)
* Along with any other food that you like that does not appear in the do not eat list
* (i.e., eat all the meat and vegetables that you like)
* Quinoa

WHY, WHY, WHY?

Firstly: Is bread killing us? Is it the latest fad? All-of-a sudden unhealthy foods that the government has engineered to keep the people down? Is it poisonous? Sorry, gang. No conspiracy here.

Bread has been around for a long, long time (about 30,000 years). So far, it hasn't decimated the human race.

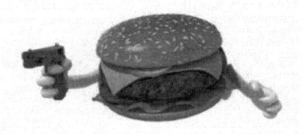

Side-note: Do you remember eating syrup sandwiches as a kid? What is a syrup sandwich you say?? When you are a kid and you're home alone after school – take a slice of Wonder bread. Pour on syrup. Lay a second slice of Wonder bread. EAT!

So no, bread isn't going to kill you but it's NOT helping you lose weight, and it's NOT helping you grow younger, either.

Now let's talk about our friend, bread:

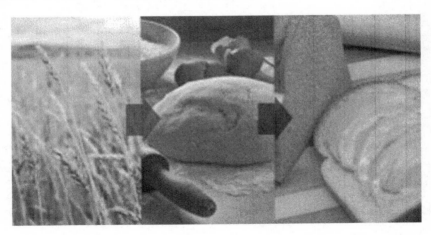

Bread is not the most naturally occurring food, right? You're never going to walk out into a field and see loaves of bread growing on a vine. It has to go through a lot of processing to

show up as the fluffy, rounded mass that we eat. Wheat →
ground to flour → + bleach (if white) → + yeast → high heat
baking.

All of that alters the Whole Food rule of eating naturally:
Watch my video here: (http://youtu.be/PMsf2UKrqr4) – this
applies to white, wheat, whole grain, pitas, all of 'em!

Bread is very bulking and filling. It's fluffy stuff that's soft and
has a lot of air in it. It's like a Nerf ball. It takes up a lot of space.
You have one tube in your body that runs from your mouth to
your pooper. That tube is narrow and that tube is elastic. The
more you clog it up with a fluffy, airy substance, the slower your
body will digest ALL of your food and the more that will expand
and add inches to your waist as it builds up.

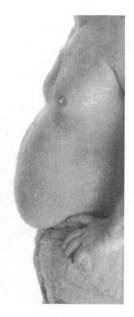

If you don't drink enough water, then it gets worse. Remember
Plaster of Paris as a kid? (No – you don't eat this one). You'd take
this white powder and mix it with water and make funny shapes
out of it and let it dry and harden? Similar to how casts for broken
bones are made. If you aren't drinking half a gallon to a gallon of
water daily (soda and coffee and energy drinks and juices are

NOT treated like water in your body – Watch my video here: (http://youtu.be/BhKD3-ty2yU) - then that chewed up bread dries up and REALLY clogs up your intestines, and that's how blockages in your digestive tract can start.

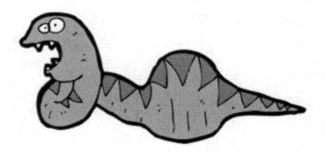

So here's the plan – Let's see if it's possible to reduce the amount of bread and other processed, fluffy, clogging carbs that we eat. So for seven days we are not going to EAT ANY BREAD!

What to Expect:

You will become very regular (2-3 bowel movements daily). You will burp less and have far less heartburn. You will notice your waist shrinking. Many of you will lose 5-10 lbs. (some have lost 20lbs+!)

"My wife has been doing zero grains for the last month and has lost 12 pounds without any exercise. If any grain is in the ingredients then she will stay away from it."

R.M.

What is the purpose?

I'm not worried about how carbohydrates are metabolized (there are carbs in apples too, but I'm not concerned about apples clogging you up). And this is not about gluten or wheat. I'm focusing on fluffy, clogging flour-based bread foods that are processed. I want you to focus on how your body starts to function, look, and feel after a few short days of temporarily eliminating bread from your diet.

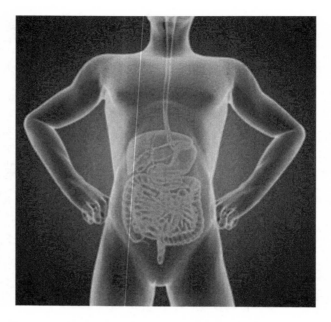

Step 1 – Join my Facebook Cleanse Support Group: www.ResetYourBody.com/SupportGroup so we can all interact and provide support, feedback, and accountability.

Step 2 – Forward this blog to your family and friends to join too! Don't try to explain it yourself (They need to see the same info you saw in order to think the same way you do.)

Tips:

- -Plan ahead. Don't end up at McDonald's.
- -And if you do, get the bunless version and a salad
- -Ask for the sandwich as a wrap instead
- -Stock up on tortilla bread at home
- -Need something to fill you up? Try beans.

Seems too simple to work, huh? I KNOW! Try it anyway. Don't take my word for it. See for yourself. Stop believing everything you hear and start doing something! I know that you can do this.

This is #3 of the 8 Challenges to Reset Your Body. And remember, when you complete this Challenge, start Challenge #4 as soon as you can.

Please share this and BE WELL.

If someone had a loaded gun to your head and demanded that you drink half your body weight in ounces of water a day, would you? If that gunman then threatened to shoot if you didn't eat a salad before every meal, would you? If he promised that he'd pull the trigger if you failed to cut out meat and breads for 5 days, would you? Yes. So we know it's physically possible.

Why don't you? Remember: You always have a choice.

My reset challenge started last week with the water and no sugar challenge. After staying consistent with my exercise routine, I'm feeling great, and it was much easier to walk away from the option of doughnuts for a quick breakfast! Progress is slow, but I'm feeling great!

RESET CHALLENGE #4: 10 DAY NO SUGAR CHALLENGE!

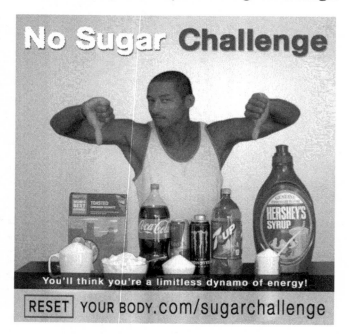

RULES FOR THE 10-DAY NO SUGAR CHALLENGE

1. Do not add sugar to any drinks or food. No sugar of any kind. (Use honey or 100% Maple Syrup only)
2. ESPECIALLY no artificial sweeteners! (Splenda, Sweet 'n Low, Equal, etc.)
3. No candies or sweets or chocolate.

4. No fast food (ten days without a Whopper won't kill you)
5. Don't use any boxed or canned foods for cooking (no frozen dinners, etc.)
6. No sodas or energy drinks (No drink with "sugar" listed on the ingredients label)
7. Drink lots of water (recommend 1/2 ounce for every pound you weigh, daily)
8. Avoid snacks or foods listing "sugar" or "corn syrup" on the ingredients label.

Update your Reset Challenge Tracking sheet

NOTE about alcohol – Alcohol itself is fine (there is no ADDED sugar in beer, wine, or gin/rum/vodka/whiskey) It's the mixers that are a no-no for this Challenge. Booze up!

What's the Purpose of The No Sugar Challenge?

This Challenge, for some of you, will be a piece of cake. You have been eating without added sugar already and you won't be fazed by this at all. Good for you! I love it. Then there are the other 90% of Americans out there. And this Challenge is going to tear you apart! The average American will consume more than 150 pounds of sugar in its various forms over the course of one year, so during this 10-day Challenge, you'll be cutting out (on average) about **4 pounds of sugar**…WOW! 4 pounds!

Five pounds every twelve days.

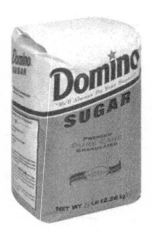

Step 1: Stop the sugar intake for a few days.

Step 2: Flush out some of the old sugar so that you can see how your body SHOULD function. It takes a lot of water to do that, so drink up! It's important to pay attention to your body so that you don't miss the lesson of this Challenge. I can't stress that enough. Body functions will change and it's not a coincidence, so stay very aware of your body for ten days!

*For the purposes of this Challenge, I'm not concerned with calories or the glycemic index. I'm concerned with a processed sweetener, a less-natural toxin that your body is reacting to. So only honey or 100% maple syrup (No Mrs. Butterworth!) for this Challenge. None of these sweeteners: SUGAR IN THE RAW, STEVIA, MOLASSES, AGAVE, etc.

Be sure to check the ingredients label on some of the food in your kitchen.

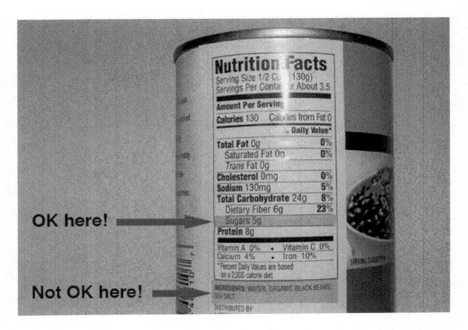

IMPORTANT: It's OK if "sugar" is listed on the nutrition facts AS LONG as it's NOT listed in the ingredients list.

Signs you might need to lower your sugar intake:

- Poor tooth health
- Low energy (dragging all day)
- Chronic pain
- Sugar cravings
- Acne
- Excessive yawning

Things to note during the Challenge: naps, energy levels, snoozing, joint pain, back pain, stomachaches, sex drive, yeast infections

What to Expect:

- More energy (no energy yo-yos),
- Less napping,
- Far easier to wake up (less drowsiness),
- Decreased chronic pain

- Crankiness
- Irritability
- Mild headaches
- Hunger

Tips:

1. Make a list of things you like to eat that don't have sugar:

- Vegetables
- Meats
- Nuts
- Seeds
- Snacks

Use lists for the various diets that are available online (or go buy the books)

2. Go shopping for these non-added sugar items.

3. Eliminate temptations. I say this after you are stocked up because it's much easier to hide or throw away food when you have something else to replace it with.

4. Try these during the Challenge to purge sugar from your body:

- Colon Cleansing
- Deep Tissue Massages
- Sauna Sweating

Sugar has been around forever. Why is it so bad now?

Let's nip this in the bud right out of the gate. Sugar is a naturally occurring nutrient (like vitamins and minerals). Sugar is found in thousands and thousands of fruits and vegetables and meats, etc. Sugar, in and of itself, is not the problem. But processed, extracted, concentrated sugar – now THAT'S THE DEVIL! That is what this Challenge is focusing on. I'll refer to it as "added sugar."

Even the best sugars you can buy (evaporated cane sugar, for example) go through a 10-15 step process:

That turns a naturally occurring sugar cane plant into table sugar.

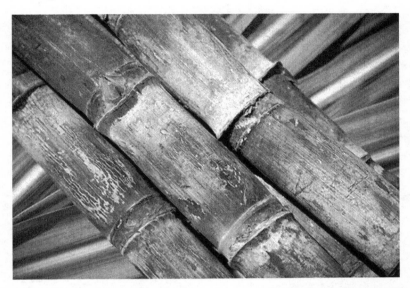

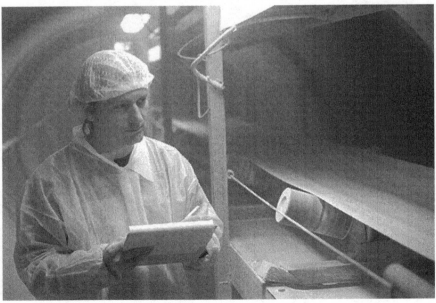

It's shredded, boiled, evaporated, strained, separated, vaporized, drained and pressed, and has chemicals added. The resulting crystals that we call sugar are no longer recognizable to your body in the normal ratio as it was in the sugar cane plant. It's literally a chemical at this point and your body treats it as such. The more you put in your body, the more will end up migrating to your body's particular weak spot and wreaking havoc (your body may just see the sugar as a threat and wrap fat around it to keep you safe). Imagine the energy your body has to constantly use (hence lowered overall energy) to clean out and remove this chemical that we keep bumping in at every meal or with every drink. Your body is working HARD!

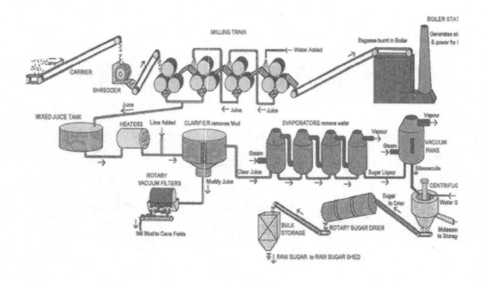

(Above) Steps to create table sugar

Artificial Sweeteners: So think about it. Splenda, Sweet 'n Low, Equal, etc. – those are 100% chemicals. The only things worse than added sugar are artificial sweeteners. Crazy, huh?! All that your body sees from those is chemical, chemical, chemical! Don't use them. EVER.

Remember:

If you eat the Standard American Diet, your body has built up a chemical dependency on sugar at this point. That's not something that you'll break overnight but you absolutely can. So don't beat yourself up if you can't last the full ten days. You can stop and restart this Challenge as many times as you need to until you make the full ten days.

Once you see how your body feels after ten days, hopefully you'll get a glimpse into your possible future. **NOTE**: To speed things up – The Veggie Cleanse and the Juice Cleanse and especially the Master Cleanse will be the most effective and dramatic ways to PURGE years and years of sugar effects and damage from your body. A Cleanse will also reset your taste buds so your cravings fade away. For now, just take it one day at time and let the compound effect of the 8 Challenges rebuild you into a new, stronger, younger you.

This is #4 of the 8 Challenges to Reset Your Body. When you complete this Challenge, start Challenge #5, The 1-Day Reset, as soon as you can.

IMPORTANT: Join my Facebook Cleanse Support Group: www.ResetYourBody.com/SupportGroup , that way we can all interact and provide support, feedback, and accountability.

Please share this and BE WELL.

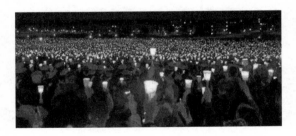

All of your 100 trillion cells are screaming for more oxygen, more water, and more waste removal. There is power in numbers. If we're in space looking at Earth, and I gave one person a candle, nothing would show to me. But if I gave a candle to everyone in your city, that city would shine from space. What if I gave a candle to everyone in America? The whole country would shine! That is what Resetting is doing to you! Drinking the water, eating the raw veggies, cutting out the bread, doing the cleanses, etc., all these things give candles to more and more of your cells. Each organ will shine better, and soon your entire body will shine better. (Strong heart cells = strong heart, etc.)

You don't have to be perfect.

Just keep making progress.

Keep improving, one cell at a time...

Ready to start lighting those candles?

PART 4:

CLEANSING YOUR BODY

Terry Givens BLOG entry Dated December 17th, 2010:

www.resetyourbody.com/why-would-someone-do-a-cleanse

Why would someone do a cleanse?

First let me be clear. All cleanses are NOT the same. There are many different types of cleanses with many different purposes. Some you only eat/drink a certain thing. Some you exclude a certain thing. Some are partial fasts. And then there are few where you fast the entire time (no food). This is specifically about a fasting cleanse…yup…no food

I remember years ago when my buddy approached me about doing the Master Cleanse. "No food for ten days!?" I yelled. I eat a full meal like every three hours. I'm from Ohio. Meat, potatoes. "No thanks, bro. I'll pass."

Then he convinced me to read the 50-page book on WHY someone would do such a fool thing and it made sense. Now I do a Master Cleanse every year – and various other simple one-day cleanses throughout the year.

(You consume enough calories in the drink so that you are NOT tired or starving to death)

It's not a diet for losing weight. You will temporarily lose weight during the cleanse, but afterwards, when your body puts the weight back on, it will be better, leaner, cleaner weight. Interestingly enough, our bodies are filled with toxins just from everyday living (food preservatives, indigestible things, chemicals…stuff). All these things and many more are still in you, slowing your body's processes down.

Changing Your Oil

It's very similar to changing your car's oil or the lint filter in your dryer, as I mentioned earlier. Your body will work more efficiently. It will process food better and need less for it to run optimally. And you will lose a ton of nasty leftover junk from your intestines (read: flatter belly and smelling better).

It's a chance to Reset your body. You never know what old festering remnant of something has been in you that is causing some sort of unwanted effect that you have slowly come to take for granted (allergies, skin conditions, joint pain).

After

Many people have had allergies disappear following a cleanse. I have friends whose lifelong snoring stopped. Joint pain has ended. I personally used to sweat a lot. After my first cleanse...no more sweating! And some have not noticed any outward improvement at all. But who's to say that their heart wasn't one french fry away from an attack? – I'm just saying.

And this is important...the benefits will come AFTER you complete the cleanse: when you are back to eating normally. Don't expect to notice improvements in yourself DURING the cleansing process. That is the clean-up phase. Inherently, during the clean-up phase of anything, things will be in disarray and transition. Be patient. Once you resume feeding your body and it starts taking advantage of the better operating equipment, THAT is when you will start noticing things.

Once toxins and waste are removed or at least reduced, your body can function much more powerfully and efficiently with much more energy. There are many types of cleanses.

- Full body cleanses
- Fasts
- Partial fasts
- Specific organ cleanses

Stay open-minded and try a few. Try to understand what the fast is accomplishing. That will help you adapt during the cleanse. Everyone's body reacts differently.

How long?

A question I get a lot is, "Why is this cleanse for ten days? Can I just do a couple of days?" Well here's a little bit of the science behind fasting. After 24-36 hours of not eating, your body switches to autophagy mode. Your body basically scavenges itself. What does it eat first? Fat, crystal deposits, toxins, cysts, lumps, garbage. The stuff you don't want. So the key is to make it past day three (the hardest day, typically) and then every day after that your cleanse is providing maximum benefit to your body.

Education

Do what I did. Download and read the book *The Master Cleanser* by Stanly Burroughs and see WHY. You might think it make sense, you might think it is dumb. But at least you decide for YOURSELF. What if a 10-day commitment could change the rest of your life? You're not getting any younger, but you can FEEL younger.

Which cleanse is right for you? Start here: www.ResetYourBody.com/detoxes

Feel free to copy that two-page blog post of mine from 2010 and give that to anyone that you would like to share the concept of cleansing with. That blog entry has led to hundreds and hundreds of people starting a new way of life that has led to more health, more energy, and more years with loved ones. It has led to new perspectives on their most valued possession – their body. So yes, you have my permission to plagiarize those two pages from my blog. Print them out, make copies. Leave them with friends, family, loved ones. Don't try to convince them to change. Don't try to explain it yourself. Don't be the pushy friend. Let them see it the same way that you saw it so that they can walk the same path and think the way you do now.

I cleanse because I don't want cancer someday. I cleanse because it makes my joints feel better, I cleanse because it keeps my muscles dense. I cleanse because it keeps my skin tight. I cleanse because it keeps my belly flat.

Cleansing

Up next are the Reset Challenges that involve cleansing. I'll be upfront and tell you right now that cleansing is how I STARTED my Reset journey years ago. I didn't have a brave and bold young man who had created gradual steps in the form of Reset Challenges to move me along. I basically STARTED with the Master Cleanse (Challenge #8) then I adopted the Water Challenge (Challenge #1) and gradually progressed through the rest as I created them. So I basically shocked my system initially, doing a major clean out to really accelerate my results. THEN I changed my lifestyle with my new, cleaner, and better working body.

Don't be 1 of the 19

What is a Cleanse?

A cleanse is defined as:

"A program of diet, herbs, and other methods of removing environmental and dietary toxins from the body."

The popularity of cleansing has grown tremendously, especially in the past five to ten years with the marked increase in obesity, cancer, heart disease, and diabetes rates. Americans are flocking to find ways to lower their chances of developing these and many other ailments.

Done safely and naturally, cleansing can be that catalyst that helps you tip the scales in favor of your body so that your body can do what it's uniquely and proficiently designed to do – grow and repair itself. But it's generally frowned on by the medical community.

Why? Is it that it's dangerous and causes death and injury? No, that prize is still held by medical drugs. (About 100,000 Americans die each year from prescription drug use.)

As I mentioned before, the medical industry and doctors in general are well intentioned (in my opinion) and they want to help people and save lives. It just so happens in our culture the medical training appears to be geared towards repair and drug use versus being geared towards prevention and natural solutions. That's all. Our experts have years and years of valuable extensive training by the drug industry on how to properly administer drugs and how to treat disease. The topic of natural and preventative treatment is just not focused on enough by the mainstream medical education system for your standard doctor to be comfortable with cleansing and natural remedies. They don't have the confidence in it and have not seen enough evidence to propose it. As a matter of fact, they have been fed enough misinformation by those entrusted to train them that the average doctor thinks that cleansing and natural remedies might even be harmful to people.

I have a high level of respect for doctors. I know for a fact that they want to help people. I'm sure that many a medical professional will get their hands on this handbook, and I know that since their professional purpose is to help, that they will at least be open to exploring avenues and tools that might help them be more effective. If nothing else, it will offer another perspective that might allow them to understand why the natural advocates think the way that they do.

This illustrates how much doctors care and want to help.

"I am a doctor. I am standing by the shore of a swiftly flowing river and hear the cry of a drowning man. I jump into the cold waters. I fight against the strong current and force my way to the struggling man. I hold on hard and gradually pull him to shore. I lay him out on the bank and revive him with artificial respiration. Just when he begins to breathe, I hear another cry for help. I jump into the cold waters. I fight against the strong current, and swim forcefully to the struggling woman. I grab hold and gradually pull her to shore. I lift her out onto the bank beside the man and work to revive her with artificial respiration. Just when she begins to breathe, I hear another cry for help. I jump into the cold waters. Fighting again against the strong current, I force my way to the struggling man. I am getting tired, so with great effort I eventually pull him to shore. I lay him out on the bank and try to revive him with artificial respiration. Just when he begins to breathe, I hear another cry

for help. Near exhaustion, it occurs to me that I'm so busy jumping in, pulling them to shore, and applying artificial respiration that I have no time to see who is upstream pushing them all in..." (Adapted from a story told by Irving Zola as cited in McKinlay, John B. "A case for refocusing upstream: The political economy of illness." In Conrad and Kern, 2nd edition, 1986, The Sociology of Health and Illness: Critical Perspectives. pp. 484-498.)

Cleanse Misconceptions

If you're anything like me, you had all sorts of preconceived notions in your head about what cleansing involved. We've all heard someone mention rumors about the process too. Here are some of the more common ones:

-"You spend all day shooting fluid and crud out of your body"
-"You will have zero energy"
-"It's just a starvation diet to temporarily lose weight"
-"It's unhealthy and unnatural and bad for your body"
-"It's only for overweight people"

Let's address these one at a time:

1. "You spend all day shooting fluid and crud out of your body"

Not true! And that's just nasty! Spending all day on the toilet and having explosive bowel movements to expel toxins is certainly not a safe, controlled cleanse. If you really think about it, that's called a flu! And, yes, that's a forced cleanse that your body does when you allow your toxic levels to become too high. Remember – you only get the flu if you need to.

A cleanse is a controlled, moderate release of toxins that is convenient and timed to allow your body to evenly and regularly control the rate of detoxing and the rate of toxin removal. Most people that undertake cleanses are regular people with regular job schedules, travel schedules, and family schedules. They have the regular demands for loved ones' celebrations and experience the same inconvenient weather deterrents that you have to deal with.

You are able to modify, tweak, shift around the timing and specifics of a cleanse to fit perfectly with your lifestyle and your demands so that you don't let your current life get in the way of your future healthier life.

2. "You will have zero energy"

Another big misconception is that you'll be so low on protein and energy and food that you will just be too darned pooped to function at work or to carry on with the high demands of a busy on-the-go person. Not true.

Firstly, there are many different types of cleanses (I'll talk about those in a bit). Many don't even involve a reduction of food intake at all. But for the few more effective cleanses that do call for a reduction or even a total eliminate of normal food intake, you will absolutely not be de-energized and dragging your body around. As a matter of fact, the vast majority of cleansers report that they feel a major BOOST in energy while cleansing. Some attribute it to their body expending less energy digesting food. Some say the herbs or liquids or foods that they do ingest during a cleanse gives them more than enough calories and protein so that they don't notice a difference at all. A huge number of cleansers have shared that they experience an amazing mental clarity while they are cleansing.

Everyone has a unique experience and the only person that can tell you how you will feel is you – when you do it. Maybe you will be one of the cleansers that continue to hit the gym every day while you are cleansing. Maybe you will be one of the cleansers that spends more time taking walks and meditating. Rest assured, you'll find out which you are.

3. "It's just a starvation diet to temporarily lose weight"

"Well, you're just losing weight because you're not eating. As soon as you start eating again you'll gain it all back and you'll have wasted your time!" Not true.

This obviously is referring to a cleanse that involves a reduction in or elimination of food. The process of cleansing is not just about reducing input. Of course, you are going to temporarily lose weight by eating far less. The magic starts to happen when you give your body a break from constantly digesting pounds and pounds of food and introduce large amounts of water into your body. The body begins to take those freed up resources and increases the river of transportation (extra water), and it cleans places that drugs and instruments can't reach. It switches from "grow" mode to "repair" mode, even if only for a day or an hour. If your body is only able to remove even the tiniest of toxins or debris or fat, your cleanse has had more of an effect than just temporary weight loss from not eating. Our job with the proper cleanse routine is to maximize the amount of clean up that your body can do with its available resources and assistance.

4. "It's unhealthy and unnatural and bad for your body"

"It's not natural to do that to your body." Not true

Let's consult our *What Would a Caveman Do* test for this one. How natural do you think it is for a caveman to spend his day constantly having access to a seemingly endless supply of filling, processed food, always walking around with a full belly from his convenient grocery store of food products?

Heck, no! Bagging deer or squirrel or meaty animal was probably (we don't know, of course, since we can't exactly go back on his timeline on Facebook to see what he did day to day) a two to three time per week treat.

He spent the bulk of his time grazing on whatever sparse plant life was palatable and a full belly was a rarity rather than a three-time-a-day occurrence. Our lifestyle now (looking back at a 200,000-year time line) is pretty darn unnatural compared with what our ancestors dealt with and what evolution has adjusted to.

The cleanses that are described in this handbook are all based on natural processes (albeit some are accelerated). There are no man-made drugs involved. They are all plant- or animal-based, things that have been around on this Earth for hundreds if not thousands of years. It's natural, it's healthy, and it's EXACTLY what your body has been doing for thousands of years.

5. "It's only for overweight people"

As we discussed earlier, fat gain and weight problems are only one way that someone's body can be affected by toxic overload. Cleansing is a cleaning process, not a weight loss diet. Certainly if you're overweight, you will lose weight if you cleanse. But even better than that, your body will decide based on its specific weaknesses and damage what parts it will clean during the process. Many athletes in fantastic physical shape swear by regular cleansing to keep their energy levels high, help their injuries heal faster, and keep their senses at their peak. Many cleansers that are models rely on their regular cleansing to keep their hair more radiant, their skin clearer, and their muscle tone perfect. Students around the world rely on their regular cleansing to sharpen their mental clarity and to ensure that they grow and develop to the fullest of their potential. How are all these things possible? Is this some sort of cure-all? Is it magic? A little bit. It's the wonderful thing that our body can do that science has not been able to explain fully. Sometimes knowing how the body works isn't as important as just knowing that it does work.

6. "It hurts"

As with anything in life, it only hurts if you're doing something wrong. I'm not a masochist, and even if you are (freak), don't expect pain from cleansing.

7. "My schedule is too crazy to do a cleanse"

Bull crap! Not true. I know people that have full time jobs (in restaurants) and have children AND they are still able to make proper sacrifices to cleanse their bodies. You do know that if you are busy you WILL certainly need to make sacrifices TEMPORARILY to Reset your health, right? It's not just going to magically fit in place. And there is never a good time to do a cleanse. Unless you are a social introvert, with no life and no friends, you may never have a five to ten day period of time in your normal life to do a cleanse. YOU WILL NEED TO MAKE TIME. And if work is the big culprit, I'll leave you with this:

Don't let a job keep you from being healthy. You're worth more than a paycheck.

8. "I eat healthily already. I don't need to cleanse"

Well, Mrs. Squeaky Guts, if you recall the toxin chart earlier, I explained how food and drink and medication are only about 30% of the toxic load that the average American is exposed to on a daily basis. Plus, our bodies are machines, and all machines make waste. Clean it up, kid!

Cleansing Benefits:

Now that we got all of the scary wrong stuff out of the way, let's talk about the cool and amazing benefits that you CAN look forward to from cleansing your body.

- Puts the body into cellular-level clean up mode
- Improves digestion
- Flattens the belly in ways sit ups cannot
- Explodes your energy
- Eliminates "incurable" illnesses
- Prevents and reverses cancer
- Allows for a less stringent diet
- Makes better skin and hair
- Eliminates foul smelling gas
- Lowers eating costs
- Eliminates cellulite
- Resets your taste buds (no cravings!)
- Helps grow back receding hair lines
- Improves eyesight
- Improves body odor
- Maintains muscle definition longer

Magic! Voodoo! This kind of talk got people burnt in the town square a few hundred years ago in old Massachusetts. Is it really magic? Nope...remember, we're simply helping to unclog our 100 trillion cells. They do the rest on their own.

Five Ways to Get Your Mind Ready:

I could name this section, "How to keep from breaking your promise to yourself," or "How to not give up on day one of a cleanse," or "How to help yourself TRULY commit to completing a cleanse." Call it what you like but this is the most important set of tips that I can give you. We've all made a promise to ourselves to make some sort of much-needed change (health, work out, relationship, savings, whatever!) but it just never happened. We either didn't start it or we did it once and then fell off the bandwagon (gyms are FULL in January and ghost towns by March.) It happens to the best of us – I've been trying to make myself wash dishes immediately after cooking for years.

I'm going to give you some super simple pointers that have helped me and hundreds of others to not only take action and START these cleanses, but to also reach our goal, cheat less, and get the full benefit that we deserve. The mind is a tricky thing. I'm going to teach you how to trick it.

1. Block off the time on your calendar

I'll say it again. There is NEVER a good time to do a cleanse. Unless you're a social derelict, you will have some sort of party or gathering or event coming up. THAT CAN'T STOP YOU! Take out your calendar and mark off the five to ten days for your cleanse. Don't let a new invitation trump your cleanse days – nothing is more important than your health and longevity! Mark it off the same way that you would mark off and plan for a wedding or a vacation.

2. Write Down Why You Are Doing It

You are about to embark on a new thing for your body. NEW. Not bad. To help yourself stay on track as you are confronted by these NEW side effects (temporary hunger, temporary healing crises, boredom, social pressure, etc.) you will need to keep that temporary emotion from taking you off your committed path. Reminding yourself WHY you're doing this in the first place will reinforce your commitment when you are weak.

Take a sheet of paper or make a note in your phone and make an exhaustive list of the benefits that you are hoping for. List how you want to feel when you reach your goal. List particular illnesses, symptoms, or problems that you'd like to be free of. List activities that you'd like to be able to enjoy if this cleanse helps. You can even write a letter to yourself. Find a picture when you were at your healthiest. Record a message to yourself. SOMETHING! This is like your half-time locker room motivation session. STAY IN THE GAME! FIGHT FOR THAT EXTRA INCH! DIG DEEP FOR AN OUNCE MORE COURAGE!

For example:

- I don't like how I look in a bikini.
- I want my knees to feel better when I walk up stairs
- I have less and less energy every year.
- I don't want to get cancer
- I'm too young to have cellulite
- I want my sweet cravings to go away
- I'm worried that I'll have a heart attack like my father and grandfather
- I want to fit into my favorite dress again
- I want a full night's sleep
- I'm sick of not being able to control my eating
- I want to set a better example for my kids
- I want to run a half marathon next year
- I don't like being judged by people when they meet me
- My friend did it; I can too!
- I don't want to be strung out on medications all my life
- I don't feel GOOD
- I'm tired of dragging around all day
- I want more energy to play with my kids/grandkids
- I've been praying. Maybe this is the answer
- I'm a fighter. I can do this!
- The drugs aren't working. I need an alternative

- I refuse to become dependent on others to live
- I don't like how I look in the mirror

Temporary pain is worth a lifetime of gain!

3. Find an Accountability Buddy

Funny thing about human beings: often we will do more for others than we'll do for ourselves. Work that to your advantage. Tell those you trust what you are doing and WHY you're doing it (NOTE: be very careful who you let into your dreams. There are those that will tear down your goals because they are afraid and they don't even know they are doing it.) Have them check in with you daily for an update. You'll find yourself staying on track simply because you know that call is coming.

Join my <u>Reset Cleanse Support Group on Facebook</u>. There are literally hundreds of accountability partners there. It's like a family. Each person is chiming in to support you and give you a pep talk if you need it – or a kick in the rear. Be vocal and share what is happening. That support will magically show up one day at the precise moment when you are at your weakest. <u>www.ResetYourBody.com/SupportGroup</u>

4. Daily Affirmations

I like to call it brainwashing. Think about it. How does the human brain learn? By repetition. Children sing the "ABC" song to themselves, actors repeat their lines in the mirror a hundred times. After a while, when you've heard it enough, you start to believe it. (Think about that when you take note of what songs you listen to repeatedly and what television programs you are exposed to on a day-to-day basis. The brainwashing can work against you too.)

5. Visualize the Process

Understanding what's happening in your body will make it a million times easier to appreciate the process instead of becoming afraid of something. Imagine if you didn't understand airplane flight: the wild turbulence during takeoff and especially mid-flight turbulence would TERRIFY you (it still does for lots of flyers anyway).

See in your mind's eye that, as your body decides which areas need healing, you may feel aches, pains, sensations. Imagine an army of cells going to work on something that needs it. If you experience nausea or cold/flu like symptoms, visualize millions of old, dormant toxins set free and your body needing to flush them out ASAP so that the clean-up process can come full circle. Imagine that someone has broken open a bag of flour and the fan is blowing that fine white powder all over the kitchen. Your body is trying to clean all that up.

WARNING!!

During your cleanse, you're going to rationalize how you've done enough, and you'll want to quit early. You'll get bored. You'll want to "reward" yourself with food. You will make the decision, literally every 60 seconds, whether to make today the last day or not. **STAY THE COURSE**. (That's just your emotions talking). Are you committed? Lean on the group. **You CAN do this.**

Things You May Notice After Cleansing

Other than a cleaner, more efficient body that processes food better, you may notice some interesting side effects that are very common.

- **More hunger** – Your body is trying to replace a few billion cells that were purged while you cleansed. It's ok to be hungry (I always am), and it's ok to eat. – EAT! Your body replaces 300 billion cells in an average day. This is your chance to give your body the best, highest quality building material to do that with. Be aware of what you put in your body during our after-cleanse hungry days!
- **Digestive issues**. During the cleanse, your body may have stopped producing its normal level of digestive enzymes and it may have washed out other beneficial bacteria in your gut during the process (I'll talk about that soon). Be

patient and follow my tips to accelerate their replacement. It's normal.

How to use this cleanse section:

Each cleanse is presented in two ways:

1. How to do the cleanse

    a. Just step-by-step instructions (each day and each time of day, etc.)

15. Why and how the cleanse works

    b. Details on the nuts and bolts

So if you just want to get down and dirty and start cleansing your little butt off, and you don't like to be bogged down with theories and how's and details, just worry about the step-by-step instructions and don't deal with the "how" and "why" section.

But if you're like me and you are the person that reads the manuals when you buy electronics, (yup, that's me), then you will find a lot of valuable information in the "why" and "how" sections that will help you to understand, maximize results, and modify for your unique needs.

Ready? Ready! Go!

RESET CHALLENGE #5: 1-DAY RESET

www.resetyourbody.com/wp-content/uploads/2013/02/1_Day_RESET_Routine.pdf

Join my Cleanse Support Group on Facebook now! Ask questions & interact. Don't do it alone!

www.ResetYourBody.com/SupportGroup

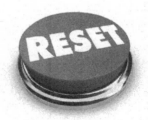

1-Day RESET Routine

RULES FOR 1-DAY RESET: FOLLOW TO THE 'T' PLEASE!

Purpose:

- You've been eating like crap lately. You had a big party weekend. You just got sick.
- Your belly is distended and that's not cute. You want something to kick-start you back into clean eating. Welcome to the 1-Day RESET!

Overview:

Do for 1 day or as many days as you feel the need.

DRINK LOTS OF WATER (1/2 your body weight in oz. daily!)

Can Eat/Drink: Any type of vegetable or fruit, nuts, yogurt, oats, beans, honey, water, coconut water, juices (AS MUCH OF THESE AS YOU LIKE!)

DON'T EAT/DRINK: Meat, breads, pastas, soda, alcohol, dairy, potatoes, processed foods (carbs slow down your pipes too much!)

Ideas:

- Eat at least **50%** of your veggies raw (don't cook it). More fiber, more alive. RAW
- Steam the veggies
- Keep apples and carrots and nuts with you at all times
- Buy big fruit platters (don't worry about the natural sugars in fruits)
- Buy pineapple & watermelon & grapes and melons and cut them up and store for the week
- Vegetarian dishes at restaurants

Things to Expect:

- Flatter stomach - lots of impacted food will loosen and go away
- Lots of peeing (washes out fat and toxins)

 DAY OF

1. First salt flush – first thing in the morning, mix 1 tablespoon of sea salt with 1 quart of lukewarm water. Drink as quickly as possible. Don't leave home for an hour. …Trust me.

2. If the salt flush doesn't work, increase the salt by 1 teaspoon each time until it does.

 BREAKFAST (**after salt flush)

1. Ginger root tea (great herb to settle digestion and to pep you up! – instructions below)
2. RESET Soup (fill your body with powerful natural antibacterial and anti-viral foods that taste great! - instructions below)
3. Eat as many fruits and veggies as you like (e.g. apples, bananas, lemons, strawberries, grapes, watermelon, pineapple.)
4. DRINK LOTS OF WATER or HERBAL TEA THROUGHOUT THE DAY – Wash out the toxins! (1/2 body weight in ounces)

 LUNCH

1. Large salad (stick with a lighter dressing, for example, Italian, vinaigrette, oil and vinegar – no creamy white dressings.)
2. Snack on carrots and apples and plums, almonds, etc.
3. DRINK LOTS OF WATER THROUGHOUT THE DAY (1/2 body weight in ounces)

NOTE: Most fast food places have $1 side salads that you can get in the drive through if you need a fast meal. You can get a tasty salad at Olive Garden – pricey but yummy!

 DINNER

1. Any type of vegetable meal (Eat as much as you want. Remember no carbs!)
2. RESET Soup (instructions below)
3. DRINK LOTS OF WATER THROUGHOUT THE DAY (1/2 body weight in ounces)

NOTE: If you can find a veggie juice bar, enjoy! Wheat grass is an acquired taste but try it out too. Otherwise, any type of veggie juice mix is perfect.

 1 hour BEFORE BED

1. Second salt flush (instructions above)
2. **Skip the second salt flush if you're RESETING for more than one day

IMPORTANT! You'll want to replace any good, beneficial bacteria lost as a side effect of the salt flushes. Keeps you from getting stomachaches and diarrhea, etc. Add one or any or all of these to your diet for the next week.

- Yogurt (with live cultures listed on the label)
- Kefir
- Sour cream
- Sauerkraut
- Pickles
- Probiotic supplements (any health store or online)

Recipes

Ginger Root Tea

Ingredients:

- Fresh Ginger Root (Reuse the same root adding 1 inch for each new serving for up to 3 days.)
- Honey and or Agave Nectar
- Water

1. Use 1 inch of ginger root for each serving of tea.
2. Cut the root into small slices
3. Low boil in water for 10 minutes
4. Add honey to taste

ENJOY!

RESET Soup

Ingredients:

- 1/4 organic red onion (major antiviral/bacterial)
- 4 cloves organic garlic (Garlic is a major antiviral/bacterial. Organic is four times more potent than non-organic. Better medicinal qualities)

1. Chop the onion and mince the garlic
1. Add to a can of healthy soup. I use chicken broth & chopped avocado.
2. Note: The soup takes away the strong taste of the onions and garlic.
3. Season to taste and add crushed red pepper (loosens mucus)
4. Bring to a boil then turn off and cover and let sit for a minute...then EAT UP!

About Reset Challenge #5

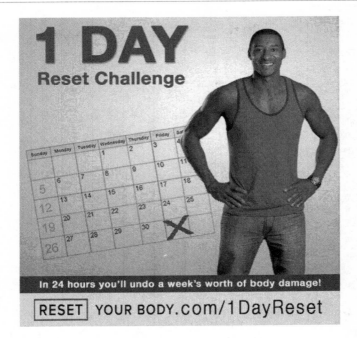

1-Day RESET

What if we could take one day, 24 hours, and undo the past week or two of bad living, or bad eating, or too much partying? That's what the 1-Day Reset is for. It's a super simple, FAST way to Reset your body and jump-start you onto the healthy train! Choo choo!

It's easy to slip up in our eating choices and our fitness goals. Can you say "vacation?" Traveling is notorious for getting people off their Reset eating habits or throwing people out of their workout routines. It's so easy to get used to doing nothing. Right?

I created this 1-Day Reset to literally kick-start my body and my energy and flush out whatever was clogging my system from the past few weeks of disciplinary digressions. It happens to the best of us.

I basically took the Veggie Cleanse (Challenge #6) and shortened it down to one day and added a few super strong antibacterial (yet tasty) concoctions to maximize the punch.

Summary of the Day:

1. Salt flush to clean out slow-moving or stalled food in your 30 feet of intestines
2. Ginger tea to fight bacterial and viral infections and improve digestion
3. Reset Soup to fight bacterial and viral infections
4. Chug water like mad all day to flush out toxins and boost energy
5. No meat or breads or pastas all day
6. No soda or energy drinks or alcohol all day
7. Another serving of Reset Soup
8. A final salt flush to get the junk out
9. Replenish any lost beneficial bacteria

Behind the Scenes:

Salt flush to clean out slow-moving or stalled food in the 30 feet of intestines

The salt flush is a salt solution that you drink first thing in the morning (before you eat anything else). It's like power washing your GI tract all the way from your mouth to your derriere! It's important to use a high quality, natural sea salt like one of these: www.redmondtrading.com/product/granular-fine/real-salt-shaker

www.healthbeyondhype.com/premier-research-labs/pink-salt-12-oz-p-64.html

www.healthbeyondhype.com/superstore/salt-fire-p-521.html

Or a high quality Himalayan salt from your local health food store. Typical table salt is so over processed, it should never be used as it can be damaging to the body.

The salt solution has the same specific gravity as your blood, so your kidneys don't need to process it, and it's not absorbed into your blood. The solution simply moves through your GI tract causing a "tidal wave" effect, pushing everything along until it comes out the other end.

NO, it doesn't hurt (why do people think all of these things hurt?)

What you can expect: Several bowel movements within 1-2 hours – STAY AT HOME!

(Speaking from experience, you do NOT want to be in the car when nature decides to call.)

Tips to make it better:

- Use warmer water to maximize results
- Squeeze some fresh lemon juice in to improve the taste 1000%.
- Try to drink the entire solution in a few minutes
- Drink another quart of water within 30 minutes afterwards
- Stay on your feet (vs. sitting or lying down) to speed up the process
- Add an additional teaspoon of salt next time if you didn't flush

If the flush didn't work:

Most people that I have worked with flush just fine. But if you didn't flush, you probably didn't follow the instructions 100% and you:

- Did not use the full quart of water
- Did not drink the full quart of solution
- Did not use at least a tablespoon of sea salt
- Did not use quality sea salt
- Took too long to drink the solution
- Ate too soon prior to flushing

Some people won't flush for a couple of reasons:

- Bowels are too clogged for the solution to make it all the way through
- Too dehydrated

- Your body, for some reason, keeps absorbing the water

Alternative if the flush didn't work:

- Oxygen colon cleansers (Mag07 or OxyFlush brands) NOT herbal colon cleansers – OXYGEN BASED colon cleansing pills

No meat, no processed carbohydrates (breads, pastas, baked goods)

The purpose here is to eat only vegetables and fruits. I want to flood your body with tons of live enzymes (the billions of tiny "soldiers" that help digest and break down the food we eat. The less you cook veggies and fruits, the more live enzymes there are) and tons of fiber to move the food from A to B. So try and eat at least half of your food raw (uncooked) on the 1-Day Reset (salads, fresh vegetables, and fruits, nuts, etc.).

We're cutting out meat and breads, pastas, baked goods, etc. for two reasons. 1) They are harder for your body to digest (energy hogs) and 2) they are more clogging. We are slowing down the intake for a day so that we can clear out old gunk and toxins.

Replenish any lost beneficial gut bacteria

One side effect of the salt flush (power washing your insides) is not only does it flush out old food, toxins and waste, it also washes out billions of the good bacteria too. A healthy person has billions of bacteria in their intestines that aid in digestion and break down and assimilate foods and nutrients. If we aren't careful, after a few salt flushes, once we go back to eating, we can have digestive issues for a while: stomach pains after eating, diarrhea, and general stomach discomfort.

The way around that is to accelerate the replacement of the good guys by:

- Eating fermented and cultured foods (yogurts, sauerkraut, pickles, kefir, etc.)

- Taking powerful probiotic supplements (1 billion+ live organisms. I know it sounds like you're putting a gaggle of alien monsters in your mouth, but don't freak out!)
- Focus on increasing these in your diet for one or two days right at the completion of your 1-Day Reset.

I just recently finished the veggie cleanse. It just had my second baby 7 months ago and am a long distant runner, but just couldn't shake the last couple pounds. It started off a little difficult, and the salt flush was utterly disgusting. After a few days, it was def better and a lot more manageable. I ended up losing more than just the last few pounds and have actually continued eating a very similar diet on a regular basis (minus the smooth move tea and salt flush). Never have I ever felt better or seen better results than I have with this cleanse. I am truly a believer.

J.A.

[Veggie Cleanse] So I'm on day 10, I feel GREAT! Less bloated, clear skin, sparkle in my eyes, I'm down 5lbs (prob mostly water?). I haven't stopped exercising (playing hours of beach volleyball, tennis, 6-mile hike yesterday, etc.).

S.S.

Finished the veggie cleanse yesterday. Lost 8lbs and feel great. More important than the weight loss is that I realized that eating a piece of fruit, almond, or veggie was not as bad as I thought. I also realized that when I think I am "starving" just grab a glass of water and it will pass.

M.S.

After treating the house for the termites, I started getting sick. I lost 20 lbs in a month, could no longer eat, could not see, had black areas in my lungs show up on x-rays with resultant asthma attacks. I used the master cleanse for 6 days. After that I was able to start eating and started regaining my health.

L.C.

RESET CHALLENGE #6: VEGGIE CLEANSE

www.resetyourbody.com/wp-content/uploads/2013/02/Veggie-Cleanse-Daily-Routine.pdf

Veggie Cleanse Daily Routine

Join my Cleanse Support Group on Facebook now! Ask questions & interact. Don't do it alone!

www.ResetYourBody.com/SupportGroup

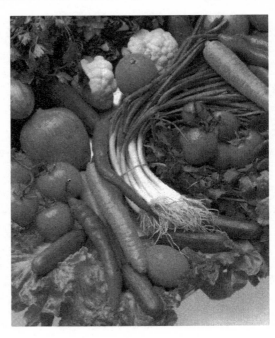

Purpose:

-Spend less energy digesting heavier foods (meats, complex carbs) and introduce a large amount of water and fruit/veggie fiber to flush out your system

Overview:

10 days of actual cleanse

Try to find someone to do the cleanse with you. The support is AWESOME!

You will have lots of energy

You will temporarily lose weight. But this is NOT a weight loss diet!

DRINK LOTS OF WATER (1/2 your body weight in ounces daily!)

Can Eat/Drink: Any type of vegetable or fruit, nuts, yogurt, oats, beans, honey, water, coconut water, juices

DON'T EAT/DRINK: Meat, breads, pastas, soda, alcohol, pastas, dairy, potatoes, and processed food

Ideas:

- Eat at least half of your veggies raw (don't cook them). More fiber, more alive. RAW
- Steam the veggies
- Keep apples and carrots and nuts with you at all times
- Buy big fruit platters
- Buy pineapple, watermelon, grapes, and melons and cut up and store for the week
- Vegetarian dishes at restaurants

DAY 1

1. Salt flush – First thing in the morning mix 1 tablespoon of sea salt with 1 quart of lukewarm water…Drink as quickly as possible. **Don't leave home for an hour…trust me.**
2. If the salt flush doesn't work increase the salt next time until it does

 BREAKFAST

1. Eat as many fruits as you like (e.g., apples, bananas, lemons, strawberries, grapes, watermelon, pineapple…)
2. DRINK LOTS OF WATER or HERBAL TEA THROUGHOUT THE DAY – Wash out the toxins! (1/2 body weight in ounces)
3. If you are light headed or hungry or anything…drink more water. It will pass.

 LUNCH

1. Large salad (stick with a lighter dressing, e.g., Italian, vinaigrette, oil and vinegar…) the waterier the better!
2. Snack on carrots and apples and plums and almonds…
3. DRINK LOTS OF WATER THROUGHOUT THE DAY (1/2 body weight in ounces)

NOTE: Most fast food places have $1 side salads that you can get in the drive through if you need a fast meal. You can get a tasty salad at Olive Garden – pricey but yummy!

 DINNER

1. Large salad
2. DRINK LOTS OF WATER THROUGHOUT THE DAY (1/2 body weight in ounces)
3. Drink a serving of laxative tea before bed.

154

NOTE: If you can find a fruit/veggie juice bar enjoy! Wheat grass is an acquired taste but try it out. Otherwise, any type of veggie juice mix is perfect.

 BEFORE BED

1. Herbal Laxative Tea from any health food store - This loosens up things inside

NOTE: If you don't have time in the morning to do the salt flush and stay home, you can do it at night an hour before you sleep.

DAY 2 – DAY 10

1. Salt flush first thing in the morning
2. Repeat Day 1 schedule
3. DRINK LOTS OF WATER or HERBAL TEA THROUGHOUT THE DAY
4. Drink a serving of laxative tea before bed.
5. You can go right into eating normally on Day 11

CONGRATULATIONS!

AFTER

IMPORTANT! You'll want to replace any good, beneficial bacteria lost as a side effect of the salt flushes. Keeps you from getting stomachaches and diarrhea, etc. Add one or any or all of these to your diet for the next week.

- Yogurt (with live cultures listed on the label)
- Kefir
- Sour cream
- Sauerkraut
- Pickles
- Probiotic supplements (any health store or online)

YOU CAN DO THIS! It's only ten days. Don't let your brain fool you into thinking that you need anything more.

Ten days of commitment could start Resetting your metabolism because you get some lame toxin out of your system.

Don'ts and Extras

This is not required reading! If you are tired of reading and understanding this thing then STOP reading and get your butt busy. BUT some of you want more details, information, tricks, and extras (like me). This is for you!

Join my Cleanse Support Group on Facebook now! Ask questions & interact. Don't do it alone!

www.ResetYourBody.com/SupportGroup/

Working out - Lots of people continue to work out while cleansing. You will have enough energy to do some light exercise. With that said, I choose to not exercise while cleansing:

1. I don't want to make myself hungry
2. We have a finite amount of energy. Why use it to build muscle for those ten days when I could have that energy to go towards cleaning up instead?
3. If I'm going to take ten days off from eating normally, I want the maximum benefits from it so I let the cleaning process take precedence.

If the salt flush doesn't work (alternatives/adjustments):

- Lemon in water makes it easier to swallow and improves taste.
- Warm water is easier too.
- Psyllium husk is an expanding colon cleanser that basically bulks up and scours the inside of your colon. Only do this if you are NOT backed up. You need to have a flowing digestion already. You can alternate every other day – salt flush one day then psyllium husks the next (mornings).

If after three days the salt flush isn't working, that means you have a blockage somewhere. Stop the salt flush and take oxygen-based colon cleanser pills for the rest of the detox (NOT herbal colon cleansers – OXYGEN-BASED colon cleansing pills [my favorites – Mag07 brand or OxyFlush brand]). Follow the instructions on the bottle.

Speeding up the process – Speed up the body's attempts to flush out and remove toxins with profuse sweating daily (hot yoga, yoga, very hot bath for 20 minutes with Epsom/bath salts, 15-20 minutes in hot sauna and or steam room). Stay hydrated!

Using your mind to deepen the detox – Envision the millions of live enzymes from the veggies bombarding old undigested food to break it down and supercharging your body's cells with tons of energy and nutrients.

Headaches/pain/flu/fever – If you experience these, it most likely means you need to drink a lot more water. For women, a half gallon of water a day, at least. For men, one gallon of water a day, at least. This is in addition to your lemonade. Your toxins are all stirred up but not getting out.

- It's normal to feel these for a half day or so. It will pass.
- If you have a lot of toxins to remove, it might take a few days.

DON'T GIVE UP. Your body isn't in pain because of lack of food. It's in pain because of released toxins. If you don't let them flush out, they will just resettle back in and continue weakening your body.

Lots of uncooked (raw) veggies – Fifty percent of your food should be uncooked. The live enzymes are the key to the magic of this detox.

Observe your body – IMPORTANT: Take inventory of your body! This might not apply until after the detox is completed and you are eating normally again.

- Skin, hair, nails, joints, breath, eyesight, etc. These things are not random. Keep track of what you notice about everything about your body. That is a sign that something was affected.

It takes more than 10 days of detoxing to remove 20–50+ years of buildup.- Every time you detox, your body will target where it sees the most need. Let your body decide what to work on next. It might take three, four, five, six, or more detoxes for your body to get to the thing that you want Reset (it took me four.)

No TV – All the food commercials will kill you. Do yourself a favor – get a book or just watch health documentaries!

Go back in time through my Cleanse Support Group:
www.ResetYourBody.com/SupportGroup

Hundreds of comments and suggestions and stories and tips and issues and highlights and lowlights from past detoxes

Effects come AFTER the detox – While you are detoxing, don't expect to see major positive changes in your body. It's like when you clean your house. Furniture is a mess, it smells like bleach. Dust is in the air. But after you're done cleaning (start to eat normally again), all the cleaned-up body systems process the nutrients better and THEN – one to two weeks after the detox – you will notice the results. Take note!

Be creative – Soups, veggie snacks, veggie options when eating out, fresh veggie juices.

Your taste buds will reset – After a detox, your taste buds will no longer need overstimulation (sugars, artificial flavorings, etc.) You will have fewer cravings for "bad" processed foods.

If you cheat, don't quit! – You WILL have a moment of weakness. Don't just stop the detox if you do. One snack does not derail the massive benefits of your detox. Wipe your mouth. Tell the support group. And get back to the plan. Your body is too damn strong to let a cheat stop you! If you can't control your stomach for ten days then who is really in charge here?

ABOUT THE RESET CHALLENGE #6: VEGGIE CLEANSE

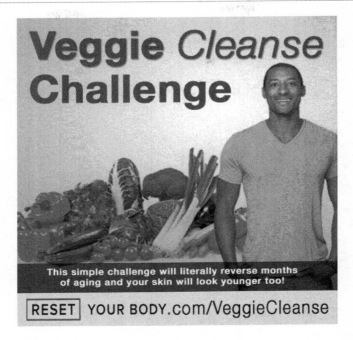

This simple challenge will literally reverse months of aging and your skin will look younger too!

RESET YOUR BODY.com/VeggieCleanse

This Challenge is really a gateway cleanse to warm up a newbie to the amazing power of detoxing.

The trickiest part about cleansing is finding the time to do it. Here's what will NOT happen: You won't wake up one day, be inspired to start your five to ten day cleanse TODAY, and find that you have ZERO social events for the week and you have no travel and no obligations. If that DOES happen, play the lotto that day, champ! Unless you live under a rock or you're a hermit or you're doing time in the pen, you will NEVER have five to ten days that happen to be perfect for doing a cleanse. There are people that have been waiting, literally, for years for the perfect time to do a cleanse. How long have you been talking about trying a cleanse? So you, my friend, will need to MAKE the time. Break out your calendar. If this is your first cleanse, plan on cleansing for five days, and then every time you Veggie Cleanse after, you add one more day until you max out at ten days. For example:

first Veggie Cleanse is five days, the next time you do it for six days, and so on, until you hit ten days.

In general, the ONLY event that should prevent you from cleansing is if you are traveling or are out of town. Salt flushes on the road are tricky, and you won't be familiar enough with whatever area you are in to find the right type of foods.

"But I have a party to attend!" – This ain't your first party and it won't be your last. A) Skip the damn party or B) show up and don't drink or eat anything other than veggies and fruits. You'll get some peer pressure from your friends to eat and drink. Here's my suggestion: Look at them closely and ask yourself, "Do I want health advice from this person?" Stick to your guns and you'll be fine with your extremely temporary sacrifice.

Want to make it even better? Recruit others to cleanse with you!

- The accountability will be priceless. When you are weak, they will help you out, and you'll help them when they slip too.
- You'll have someone to complain to.
- You'll have more fun.
- You can even have everyone in your office at work participate!
- Join my Reset Cleanse Support Group online for tons of support.

Prepare yourself for how your body will react as it starts flushing out and eliminating years of built up toxins. Some of you will do this Veggie Cleanse and it won't faze you one bit. Maybe you've been eating clean for years or you have cleansed most of your toxins out already, so these days will fly by and you won't even notice much. Then there are the other 95% of you out there.

You folks who, by no fault of your own, have been eating a normal Standard American Diet. Why wouldn't you? So is 95% of the population. Americans eat American food, obviously. As you progress through this simple cleanse of eating live vegetables and triggering your body's natural internal clean-up mechanism, you may feel some unpleasantness as your body finally gets an opportunity to get the garbage out.

Signs That You Are Detoxifying:

- Sluggishness
- Hunger and cravings
- Sensitive skin
- Cold and flu-like symptoms
- Temporary skin rashes or discolorations
- Slight fever

"What the hell?!" you say. Why on God's green earth would someone put up with all that, on purpose? I'll tell you why. Because you're full of 20, 30, 40, 50+ years of every chemical used to grow and preserve food that you've eaten. You have impacted fecal matter in your intestines that have been cooking at 98 degrees for years. You have drugs and medication that are literally part of you at a cellular level. (What goes into your mouth is used as the building blocks to create your body, every day.)

It doesn't mean that you're dying, or that you're making yourself sick if you feel these symptoms during a cleanse. All you're doing is removing meats and breads and pasta from your diet and eating lots more vegetables and fruits. Why on Earth would that simple, natural change make you sick? It's just food, right? It's not like you injected yourself with a poison or a strain of germ. That's the kind of thing that will make you sick. The act of purging your body of poisons and germs will too.

Summary of the Day:

1. Salt flush to clean out slow-moving or stalled food in the 30 feet of intestines
2. Chug water like mad all day to flush out toxins and boost energy
3. No meat or breads or pastas all day
4. No soda or energy drinks or alcohol all day
5. Laxative tea before bed

6. AFTER: Replenish any lost beneficial bacteria
7. Eat BETTER!

Behind the Scenes:

Laxative Tea

The laxative tea helps to accelerate the removal of old fecal matter from your body. You take the tea at night, and its job is to loosen up years of impacted food, like Drano down a clogged sink. Some of that food has been in there so long, and it's so dried out, it is literally as hard as a rock, and it will take continuous attempts to loosen it up and break it free. Be patient! In the mornings, you do the salt flush and it pushes out anything that was loosened up. Repeat the cycle each day during the cleanse. Depending on how much you had in you, you'll notice some pretty darn significant slimming of your waist.

Salt flush to clean out slow-moving or stalled food in the 30ft of intestines

The salt flush is a salt solution that you drink first thing in the morning (before you eat anything else). It's like power washing your GI tract all that way from your mouth to your derriere! It's important to use a high quality, natural sea salt as shown below:

- http://bit.ly/1cqH69A
- http://bit.ly/1ImRQqE
- http://bit.ly/1KDBpbx

Or a high quality Himalayan salt for your local health food store. Typical table salt is so over processed, it should never be used as it can be damaging to the body.

The salt solution has the same specific gravity as your blood, so your kidneys don't need to process it, and it's not absorbed into your blood. The solution simply moves through your GI tract causing a "tidal wave" effect, pushing everything along until it comes out the other end.

NO, it doesn't hurt (why do people think all of these things hurt?)

What you can expect: several bowel movements within 1-2 hours – STAY AT HOME!

(Speaking from experience, you do NOT want to be in the car when nature decides to call.)

Tips to make it better:

-   Use warmer water to maximize results
-   Squeeze some fresh lemon juice in to improve the taste.
-   Try to drink the entire solution in a few minutes
-   Drink another quart of water within 30 minutes afterwards
-   Stay on your feet (vs. sitting or lying down) to speed up the process
-   Add an additional teaspoon of salt next time if you didn't flush

If the flush didn't work:

Most people that I have worked with flush just fine. But if you didn't flush: you didn't follow the instructions 100% or you:

-   Did not use the full Quart of water
-   Did not drink the full Quart of solution
-   Did not use at least a tablespoon of sea salt
-   Did not use quality sea salt
-   Took too long to drink the solution
-   You ate too soon prior to flushing

Some people won't flush for a couple of reasons:

-   Bowels are too clogged for the solution to make it all the way through
-   Too dehydrated
-   Your body, for some reason, keeps absorbing the water

Alternative if the flush didn't work:

-   Oxygen colon cleansers (Mag07 or OxyFlush brands) NOT herbal colon cleansers – OXYGEN BASED colon cleansing pills

- **No meat, no processed carbohydrates (breads, pastas, baked goods)**

The purpose here is to eat only vegetables and fruits. I want to flood your body with tons of live enzymes (the billions of tiny "soldiers" that help digest and break down food we eat. The less you cook veggies and fruits, the more live enzymes there are) and tons of fiber to move the food from A to B. So try and eat at least half of your food raw (uncooked) on the 1-Day Reset (salads, fresh vegetables and fruits, nuts, etc.).

We're cutting out meat and breads, pastas, baked goods, etc. for two reasons. 1) They are harder for your body to digest (energy hogs) 2) they are more clogging. We are slowing down the intake for a day so that we can clear out old gunk and toxins.

Replenish any lost beneficial gut bacteria

One side effect of the salt flush (power washing your insides) is not only does it flush out old food, toxins and waste, it also washes out billions of the good bacteria. A healthy person has billions of bacteria in their intestines that aid in digestion and break down and assimilate foods and nutrients. If we aren't careful, after a few salt flushes, once we go back to eating we can have digestive issues for a while: stomach pains after eating, diarrhea, and general stomach discomfort.

The way around that is to accelerate the replacement of the good guys.

- Eating fermented and cultured foods (yogurts, sauerkraut, pickles, kefir, etc.)
- Taking powerful probiotic supplements (1 billion plus live organisms. I know it sounds like you're putting a gaggle of alien monsters in your mouth, don't freak out!)
- Focus on increasing these in your diet for one to two days right at the completion of your 1-Day Reset.

Hallelujah!!! I've been waiting patiently for day 4 to arrive!!! I was actually sick the weekend before the master cleanse began so I was very apprehensive to move forward because I already felt horrible! But I did! And honestly...I felt like absolute CRRAAPPP for 3 days straight...every horrible symptom we were told we might experience...I DID! Then finally, this morning, I woke up with no headache, no stomachache, my body no longer feels like it's been hit by a truck and actually feeling somewhat normal, with a lot more energy!!!

M.P.

Even though I only did 5 days on the juice fast I feel like I have really improved my digestion! Great experience for me!

W.B.

I am the guy that lost 40 lbs last year juicing(it took just 90 days). Don't worry I had real food during the 90 days. I started off with a 5 day juice cleanse followed by 90 days of juicing/eating healthy . I have had 2 back surgeries in 2 years so I was not able to exercise AT All! So keep up the hard work and realize that the nutrition alone is enough to help you lose all the weight you want!

S.B.

I spoke with Terry today and he mentioned there was a type 1 diabetic in the group. I'd love to connect to exchange experiences. End of Day 2 of 70% Juice / 30% Raw Veggie Cleanse. My blood sugar between 100 and 120 despite drinking juices and cutting down on insulin in half. This is my 2nd time and yet again amazing results.

K.S

Day 9, I just weighed myself and I'm down 13 lbs since starting this! I plan to continue juicing for 30 days and just allow myself one raw meal a day. I want to be the healthiest me I can be.

G.L.

RESET CHALLENGE #7: JUICE CLEANSE

Juice Cleanse Daily Routine

www.resetyourbody.com/wp-content/uploads/2013/03/Juice-Cleanse-Daily-Routine.pdf

Join my Cleanse Support Group on Facebook now! Ask questions & interact. Don't do it alone!

www.ResetYourBody.com/SupportGroup

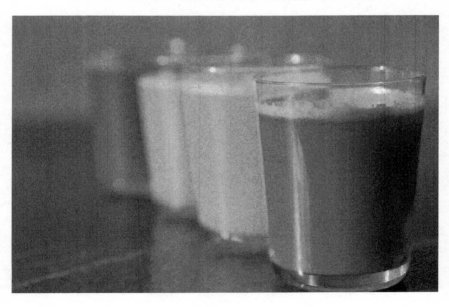

RULES FOR JUICE CLEANSE: This is the just the super short HOW TO guide. It is NOT the theory and it is not "how this cleanse" works document. This is for those people that wouldn't read that anyway. These are your marching orders. FOLLOW TO THE 'T' PLEASE!

Purpose:

- Spend less energy digesting heavier foods (meats, complex carbs).
- Avoid digestive sluggishness by absorbing large amounts of nutrients from juice directly into your bloodstream.

Overview:

- 10 days of actual fasting (**5 days for first timers**)
- 1-2 days to ease out of the cleanse
- Total of 12 days
- Try to find someone to do the cleanse with you. The support is AWESOME!
- You will have lots of energy
- You will temporarily lose weight. But this is NOT a weight-loss diet!
- DRINK LOTS OF WATER!

Can Drink

- * Fresh fruit and vegetable juice (fresh is best.)
- * Best – drink within 20 minutes of juicing (live enzymes start to die after juicing)
- * Next best – seal in airtight container and drink within 24 hours of juicing
- * Next best (in a pinch) – natural juices like Naked, Odwalla, V-8, etc.
- * Water, herbal tea, and unflavored coconut water are allowed throughout the day

DON'T Drink

- Sodas, alcohol, coffee.
- Avoid pre-packaged juices (pasteurization and storage = little if any nutrition)

Ideas

- Find a local juice bar if you're on the go
- Fresh OJ
- Organic produce is far better and worth it but use whatever you have.
- Add fresh peppers (jalapeno, etc.) or cayenne powder or other hot sauce to juice to help loosen mucus during the Juice Cleanse
- You will become very regular (3-4 times per day...GET IT OUT!)
- More frequent urination
- Maybe temporary minor headaches or flu like symptoms (when you stir up toxins to remove them you can feel it)
- Flatter stomach – lots of impacted food will loosen and go away

Track your progress:

- Your Start Date:
- Start Weight:
- Your End Date:
- End Weight:

One day before the Juice Cleanse

- Go shopping for your supplies at any health food store (Sprouts, Trader Joes, etc.)

NEEDED:

- Juicer (Not a blender. They are very different.)
- Psyllium husk
- Any brand of natural laxative tea

- Any brand of herbal tea
- Three days of fruits and vegetables

***be sure to include dark green leafy greens. 80% veggie, 20% fruit

Daily Routine (Days 1 – 10)

1. Salt flush – wake up and mix 1 tablespoon of sea salt with 1 quart of lukewarm water…Drink as quickly as possible. Don't leave home for an hour…trust me ;-).
2. Plan to drink 3-5 juices per day, 16-20 ounces each spread throughout the day (80% veggie, 20% fruit).
3. Drink AT LEAST 64 ounces of water in addition to juice. The more the better!
4. Drink a cup of natural laxative tea before bed.

Ease off day (Day 11)

1. Raw fruit for first half of the day.
2. Raw vegetables (and salad) for second half of the day.

AFTER

IMPORTANT! You'll want to replace any good, beneficial bacteria lost as a side effect of the salt flushes. Keeps you from getting stomachaches and diarrhea, etc. Add one or any or all of these to your diet for the next week.

- Yogurt (with live cultures listed on the label)
- Kefir
- Sour cream
- Sauerkraut
- Pickles
- Probiotic supplements (any health store or online)

Don'ts and Extras

This is not required reading! If you are tired of reading and understanding this thing then STOP reading and get your butt busy. BUT some of you want more details, information, tricks, and extras (like me). This is for you!

Join my Cleanse Support Group on Facebook now! Ask questions & interact. Don't do it alone!

www.ResetYourBody.com/SupportGroup/

Working out - Lots of people continue to work out while fasting. You will have enough energy to do some light exercise. With that said, I choose to not exercise while fasting:

1. I don't want to make myself hungry
2. We have a finite amount of energy. Why use it to build muscle for those ten days when I could have that energy to go towards cleaning up instead?
3. If I'm going to take ten days off from eating normally, I want the maximum benefits from it so I let the cleaning process take precedence.

If the salt flush doesn't work (alternatives/adjustments)

- Lemon in water makes it easier to swallow and improves taste.
- Warm water is easier too.
- Psyllium husk is an expanding colon cleanser that basically bulks up and scours the inside of your colon. Only do this if you are NOT backed up. You need to have a flowing digestion already. You can alternate every other day – salt flush one day then psyllium husks the next (mornings).
- If after three days the salt flush isn't working, that means you have a blockage somewhere. Stop the salt flush and take oxygen-based colon cleanser pills for the rest of the detox (NOT herbal colon cleansers – OXYGEN-BASED colon cleansing pills [my favorites – Mag07 brand or OxyFlush brand]). Follow the instructions on the bottle.

Speeding up the process – Speed up the body's attempts to flush out and remove toxins with profuse sweating daily (hot yoga, yoga, very hot bath for 20 minutes with Epsom/bath salts, 15-20 minutes in hot sauna and or steam room). Stay hydrated!

Too many fruit juices will get you bloated – Stick to 80% veggies and 20% fruits just to even the flavor out. My favorite? The Reset Juice: Kale, Carrot, Lemon, Apple.

Using your mind to deepen the detox –

Envision billions of live enzymes from the juice as tiny soldiers digesting all the old food in your gut and supercharging your body's cells with tons of energy and nutrients!

Headaches/pain/flu/fever – If you experience these, it most likely means you need to drink a lot more water. For women, a half gallon of water a day, at least. For men, one gallon of water a day, at least. This is in addition to your lemonade. Your toxins are all stirred up but not getting out.

- It's normal to feel these for a half day or so. It will pass.
- If you have a lot of toxins to remove, it might take a few days. DON'T GIVE UP. Your body isn't in pain because of lack of food. It's in pain because of released toxins. If you don't let them flush out, they will just resettle back in and continue weakening your body.

Fresh juice only – For full benefit, you want to try to drink the juice no more than 20 minutes after juiced. Remember how an apple browns after you bite it? Those are enzymes dying. Drinking your juice within 20–60 minutes is optimal. Same day is next best. Next day or bottled juices are last place for live soldiers!

Observe your body – IMPORTANT: Take inventory of your body! This might not apply until after the detox is completed and you are eating normally again.

-Skin, hair, nails, joints, breath, eyesight, etc. These things are not random. Keep track of what you notice about everything about your body. That is a sign that something was affected.

Takes more than 10 days of detoxing to remove 20–50+ years of buildup - Every time you detox, your body will target where it sees the most need. Let your body decide what to work on next. It might take three, four, five, six, or more detoxes for your body to get to the thing that you want Reset (it took me four.)

No TV – All the food commercials will kill you. Do yourself a favor – get a book or just watch movies!

Go back in time through my Cleanse Support Group: www.ResetYourBody.com/SupportGroup

Hundreds of people and pages of comments and suggestions and stories and tips and issues and highlights and lowlights from past detoxes.

Effects come AFTER the detox – While you are detoxing, don't expect to see major positive changes in your body. It's like when you clean your house. Furniture is a mess, it smells like bleach. Dust is in the air. But after you're done cleaning (start to eat normally again), all the cleaned-up body systems process the nutrients better and THEN – one to two weeks after the detox – you will notice the results.

Your taste buds will reset – After a fast, your taste buds will no longer need overstimulation (sugars, artificial flavorings, etc.) You will have fewer cravings for "bad" processed foods!

If you cheat, don't quit! – You WILL have a moment of weakness. Don't just stop the detox if you do. One snack does not derail the massive benefits of your detox. Wipe your mouth. Tell the support group. And get back to the plan. Your body is too damn strong to let a cheat stop you! If you can't control your stomach for ten days. Then who is really in charge here?

About Reset Challenge #7 Juice Cleanse

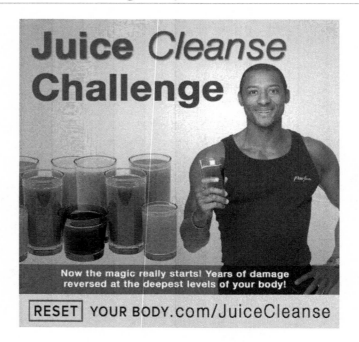

Now we're getting into the good stuff! At this point, you should have incorporated the first four Reset Challenges into your day-to-day lifestyle. You should be drinking half an ounce per pound of water every day, eating two to three salads per day, avoiding breads and pastas, and eliminating added sugars from your diet.

Depending on your particular body (two-thirds of Americans are overweight, so I shall assume), you hopefully have lost 5-10 pounds from each Challenge. What have you noticed about your body as you progressed through each of these simple yet super impactful changes in your lifestyle? Bowel movements that are more regular? More energy? Better skin? Less chronic pain? Less snoozing when the alarm goes off? Reduction in some other chronic illness symptoms? An increase in your clothes shopping budget, as you've had to buy smaller and smaller clothing sizes? Make a list in your notepad if you haven't been tracking it already!

So at this point, it's time to take the gloves off! You believe this stuff works now, right? It's not just a fluke. What you've been systematically doing is 1) providing more oxygen to your cells, 2) providing more water to your cells, and 3) hypercharging your body's waste removal systems. Now we're going to accelerate the process!

This Juice Cleanse is a safe, controlled, hypereffective method to remove years of toxic residue and impacted fecal matter and bombard your cells with concentrated nutrients from juice directly into your bloodstream. And we do all of this while not eating any solid food. That's correct. It's a fast!

"This doesn't seem very natural, Terry. Cavemen never juiced vegetables! What gives here?" Well smarty-pants, you're absolutely right. It's not natural for cavemen to do juice fasts, nor is it natural to be exposed to the extreme levels of toxic load that we are exposed to today (see the chart from the Toxin chapter) with food additives and air pollutants and water treatment, etc. Remember, Resetting is about undoing years and years of toxic damage to the body. We're in major CLEAN-up mode here. We're trying to undo years of damage in a few months' time. With all of that unnaturally high exposure for all these years, it's okay to swing the pendulum the other way, TEMPORARILY, to clean things out. Get it? GOOD!

Summary of a Day:

1. Salt flush to clean out slow-moving or stalled food in your 30 feet of intestines
2. Chug water like mad all day to flush out toxins
3. Drink three to five glasses fresh vegetable juice throughout the day
4. No solid food
5. Laxative tea before bed
6. Replenish any lost beneficial bacteria

Behind the Scenes:

See previous chapter about salt flush.

The magic of concentrated vegetable juice

So we're all agreed that eating more vegetables and fruits is better for your overall health. So why not just eat tons of vegetables and fruits instead of taking all of the juice out and discarding the very valuable fiber? I'll tell you why.

It's a pretty well-known fact that due to poor crop rotation and an overuse of chemical and artificial fertilizers, our soil has grown progressively more and more depleted of nutrients over the years. Since that is the food that plants eat, the plants that we grow to eat have become less nutritious as well. There are those that say we would need to eat five apples today to equal the nutritional value of one apple that our grandparents ate. So now the question is, who has time to eat five damn apples?

Juicing is a great way to increase our nutritional intake from vegetables and fruits without having to eat our body weight in plants all day long.

Can I use a blender?

Let's say you're like 90 percent of Americans and you don't have a juicer in your kitchen. The next question is, "Can I use a blender or a Ninja or a NutriBullet or a Vitamix and have the same results on the Juice Cleanse?" The super strong ones can turn those vegetables into liquid. That's good enough, right?

NOPE.

Remember all that fiber and pulp that is removed when juicing? The removal of that excess material is what allows the juice to bypass the normal digestion process. Juice is mainlined straight into your bloodstream. Let's say after years of damage, your body doesn't digest and pull enough nutrients from food that you eat. The last thing that you want to do is hinge your healing on your less-than-perfect digestion. We need something that is going to bypass that damaged system altogether and get the cure into your body's cells where it's needed.

That's not to say that blending vegetables is a waste of time. It's SUPER beneficial but not for a juice cleanse. Use that Ninja or Bullet along with your normal diet to supplement your body with energy-giving liquefied veggies. During the cleanse, stop by a juice bar three or four times a day and pay $5 for someone else to juice it up for you. GOT IT?

What about the sugar in fruits and fruit juice?

Let's touch a bit on fruits and sugars. Sugar itself is not the devil (contrary to popular belief). Sugar is a naturally occurring substance. It's just a type of carbohydrate. Sugar is found in the tissue of most plants. Sugar has been around for billions of years. So sugar is part of most plants, right? Do we see plant-eating animals running around with diabetes and rampant obesity? Nope. The issue that we as humans have with sugar is that we isolate and concentrate sugar with a 12-step process that just gives us too much of a good thing in a supercharged form and, nowadays, it's in almost all boxed/canned/processed food...TOO MUCH! Naturally occurring sugars that are in the fruit juice that we consume while juicing aren't anywhere near the concentrations we get when we consume granulated, processed sugar. BUT, after years of sugar abuse (like most Americans have been exposed to), we do want to be mindful how much we take in when we're juicing.

Generally speaking, green leafy vegetables will provide the most beneficial nutrients for your Juice Cleanse. With that said, all types of vegetables and fruits will provide different levels and types of unique healing and nourishing benefits, so shoot for diversity in your juicing but lean towards green leafy veggies.

Juice recipes and mixing tips:

So what should you put in your juice?

Here are my three simple juice recipe rules:

- It should be roughly 80% vegetables and 20% fruits
- Include a green leafy vegetable
- Start with a base of carrots or celery
- That's it! I'm a simple guy. I have simple rules

You do not need to break out a math equation to figure this out. The point is, the vast majority should be vegetable then you add some fruit for flavor. NOTE: If you reverse this ratio and your juices are mostly fruit juice, you'll start to notice that you will feel bloated or have an upset stomach.

I usually throw in all my vegetables then I add a green apple and squeeze a whole lemon in to smooth out the flavor...BOOM!

Start with a base of carrots or celery

Some vegetables don't release as much juice as others. The precious green leafy vegetables are on the low end of the juice-abundance spectrum. It's hard to fill up a glass with just green leafy veggies, BUT the green juice is so packed with nutrients, so that's okay.

That's why we start with a base vegetable that releases lots of juice (to fill up our glass) and to provide lots of nutrient-packed juice to give our bodies that fuel and energy they will need to keep going all day long.

Carrots and celery are the juice kings that you will choose from as the base for your juices. I personally don't use recipes when I juice. I just grab a base, then chuck in some green leafy veggies, maybe some other veggie that caught my eye, then top it off with a green apple and a squeezed lemon.

Example:

THE RESET JUICE

- [Base] Carrots
- [Green] Spinach
- [Fruit] 1 Green apple and squeezed lemon
- OR
- [Base] Celery
- [Green] Kale
- [Other] Beet
- [Fruit] 1 Green apple and squeezed lemon

NOTE: I don't put my lemon through the juicer. I simply cut it in half and squeeze it into my drink and stir. Try whatever you prefer.

How much?

Three 15 ounce to 20 ounce glasses of fresh juice per day will be enough for the vast majority of people...REALLY! It doesn't sound like much, but you'll be very surprised how little of this highly potent juice you need to keep up with your normal activities. I'm 6' 2" and 200lbs and I eat a good amount of food normally. But I can make it just fine on three or four glasses of juice per day during a Juice Cleanse.

Let's rapid fire a few issues that you might have and see if we can make this process easier for most of you:

"I don't have a juicer"

Good! Then you can do what I do – find a juice bar near you and buy your fresh juice two to three times per day.

You'll be surprised to find, once you start to actively look around or search the Internet, that you have a juice bar near you in most major cities. (The Whole Food grocery chains all have juice bars.)

"I don't have juice bars in my town"

That's totally possible in smaller towns and especially outside of California. Answer: Buy a juicer.

You can pick up a good juicer online or at a major mall. You can pay anywhere from $50 to as much as $1000. I recommend spending around $150 to get a quality juicer that can handle hard fruits and veggies without having to pre-chop them. And that price range should get you one that is easier to clean. (I'm a bachelor and cleanup was my biggest concern with juicing at home.) My $150 Breville Juice Fountain plus has lasted me seven years, is super easy to clean, and can handle whole apples and large, hard fruits and veggies. It's served me well.

"I don't like the taste of vegetable juice/vegetables"

Surprisingly enough, there are MANY of you out there. Plant haters! The good news is that most people are able to switch that distaste off and become avid vegetable and juice lovers. The issue in most of those cases has been one of two things:

1. Years of eating processed, overly sugared foods led to over stimulation of the taste buds/chemical residue in the body that impairs normal tasting. *Solution* – one of the byproducts of fasting cleanses is that it resets your taste buds. The temporary relative understimulation of the taste buds combined with the body's removal of addictive chemical residue, partially or fully corrects your taste buds so you can enjoy good old naturally flavored foods. (Take advantage of these new taste buds after your cleanse. Eat clean and stay away from sugary junk foods and you will have less issue with junk cravings.)

2. Only eating conventionally grown, bland, flavorless, weakened, less-potent vegetables doesn't get anyone's mouth too excited. As I mentioned before, avoiding pesticide residue on foods is NOT my number one reason for eating organic foods. The main reason I eat organic is because NON-organic food are less healthy. Plants grown with chemical fertilizers and sprayed with pesticide chemicals and prematurely ripened using gases are less mature, less nutritious, less flavorful, less vibrant, less energetic, and less healthy. It's common sense. Our food is what IT eats too. That reduction of flavor in fruits and veggies that has been occurring with conventionally grown food in America for the past 60 years has most grocery store produce tasting like cotton.

I lived in Sweden for four months. After returning to America, I was dumbfounded how bland and flavorless our food is here in the States. My poor taste buds were very disappointed when eating out for a couple of months. Most European nations have outlawed over 150 chemicals additives that are legal AND commonly used in foods here in America. Bland food needs something to make it taste better! Many larger American food corporations actually sell the same food abroad but they first reformulate it and remove the chemicals for overseas consumers…CRAZY, HUH?

Healing Crisis

Be sure to read my chapter about healing crisis, so that you understand what to expect to feel.

Ease Off Day

Before you run and eat a tub of fried chicken and a hot fudge brownie sundae as your first after-cleanse meal, let's talk about the all-essential Ease Off Day. Why do you need it? If you don't ease off the cleanse properly, you run the risk of having stomach aches or diarrhea once you start eating again.

What the heck is all that about? Well, for the past few days your body hasn't needed to digest any solid, dense foods, so it has slowed down its production of digestive enzymes. Without those enzymes, your body won't be able to properly digest that bacon cheeseburger and apple pie just yet.

One of two things will happen: 1) It will sit in your belly like a log. You will get a major stomachache since there aren't enough enzymes to break it down yet. Or 2) it will make it past your stomach okay (yay!) but it won't be broken down by your out-of-practice digestive tract. Then starts the diarrhea or the hemorrhoids – NASTY, HUH?

Since we obviously don't want that, we take a day to help build up those digestive enzymes. A half a day of raw fruit followed by a half a day of raw vegetables will do just the trick to let your body ramp up that enzyme production.

Example Ease Off Day:

Breakfast – fruit salad or other fruits
Lunch – vegetable Salad with avocado
Dinner – vegetable Salad
Snacks – baby carrots, cucumbers, grapes, apple

Replenish any lost beneficial gut bacteria

One side effect of the salt flush (power washing your insides) is not only does it flush out old food, toxins, and wastes, it also washes out billions of the good bacteria. A healthy person has billions of bacteria in their intestines that aid in digestion and break down and assimilate foods and nutrients. If we aren't careful, after a few salt flushes, once we go back to eating, we can have digestive issues for a while: stomach pains after eating, diarrhea, and general stomach discomfort.

The way around that is to accelerate the replacement of the good guys.

- Eating fermented and cultured foods (yogurts, sauerkraut, pickles, kefir, etc.)
- Taking powerful probiotic supplements (1 billion plus live organisms. I know it sounds like you're putting a gaggle of alien monsters in your mouth. Don't freak out).
- Focus on increasing these in your diet for one to two days right at the completion of your Juice Cleanse.

The Master Cleanse changed my life. After 10 days of drinking only lemonade without any solid food I now have more energy, feel healthier, and can eat vegetables for the first time in over 20 years

J.O.

After I was diagnosed and treated for breast cancer, I developed asthma. Those conditions had me on 13 different medications. I felt very unhealthy. I was open to something different. I did the Master Cleanse for 10 days. During it I coughed up tons of mucus, had pain in my sinuses, kidney pain, and a cracking in my lungs…apparently that was a healing because my asthma was gone by the end!

P.S.

Last year was my first Master Cleanse and since then I have not had allergies like I have in the past!

N.S.

Finishing up day 10 on the Master cleanse. I've lost 10lbs and my energy is way up. Thank you everyone on this support group for pushing me to keep going when I wanted to quit on day 5.

K.F.

I DID IT!!!!!!!!!!10 DAY MASTER CLEANSE DONE!!!!!!
Never been so proud of my willpower to not eat junk food and I feeeel amazing!!

J.M.

My energy has been really good the last few days & definitely notice a difference in sinus congestion/pressure as well. I'd had sinus issues for years, to the point my doc recommended surgery, but the cleanse has helped. It's not 100% better, but there has been an improvement

A.H.

Finished! 7 days of Master Cleanse + 3 days of juice detox. Lost 16 lbs of bear fat and 40 years of sludge. I feel fantastic. Physically clean, mentally clear. Like I just returned from a satisfying vacation: Reset! Thank you all the rest whose posts kept me on track. Will def do it again

S.Z.

After two pregnancies I always had that belly pooch that stuck out. I was never overweight but just 10 pounds over my target weight no matter how hard I worked out. It was really frustrating! I noticed right away during the cleanse that my belly really flattened up. I realized that I was really addicted to carbs and sugar and that was what was holding me up. After the cleanse, I didn't crave carbs at all and I remember trying ice cream and it was so sugary and disgusting. I think it's a great way to reset your body to healthier cravings and feel better overall. I love it!

B.L.

I know my cleanse is working because yesterday I was EXTREMELY SORE ALL OVER. My damn triceps were even sore! From what I read, that's totally normal and expected. The soreness is from all the toxins loosening up in your body. I do my salt wash at night so most of those painful/achy toxins were gone by this morning

H.J.

Day 4: down 8lbs so far! Blood pressure: 147/113. Blood sugars were a little higher than day 3, but still not too shabby. I had blood tests done before this cleanse to test a lot of different stuff but mostly to see what my kidney function was before and after and also my A1C (blood sugar average for 3 months) my kidney function starting was 30% (yikes) & A1C was 12.7 (giving my average blood sugar for 3 months in the 300's) really bad!

G.L.

What a day 3 for me yesterday. Borderline Migraine all day with nausea late in the day culminating with a pullover on the drive home to throw up twice on some poor guy's building. Then Epsom salt bath when I got home followed by more water and a few projectile vomits (luckily I was close to the bathroom, I only missed a little), then a two hour nap. I felt a bit better after that with no migraines, however I think I sprained my tongue in the process…, yes, you heard that right… I was a bit concerned because it looked like I might have had some blood come up. (Wow, what am I eliminating…) Whatever it is, I'm glad I don't have it anymore. Woke up this morning on Day 4 for me and I feel a thousand times better and starting to pass some really strange colors (I'll leave it at that)

C.Y.

It has been an amazing 5 days of doing the Master Cleanse, lost 10lbs & 2 inches on my waist, my acne cleared up and joints feel better! I look forward to the next time, thank you for every ones support. Each one of you have inspired me!

J.P.

After treating the house for the termites I started getting sick. I lost 20 lbs in a month, could no longer eat, could not see, had black areas in my lungs show up on x-rays with resultant asthma attacks. I used the master cleanse for 6 days. After that I was able to start eating and started regaining my health.

L.C.

The first time I decided to do the master cleanse I felt peer pressured because a group of people at the gym were trying to convince me to join them. I didn't know much about it so I went to Henry's and bought the little yellow book. After I read the benefits of doing a master cleanse and how all religions and other cultures around the world usually do some sort of a fast every year, I decided to jump on the bandwagon. (Even though I wasn't 100 percent sold on it). It was fairly easy to follow the directions, there wasn't that many ingredients. I found it easiest for me to bring a large 1-gallon container with the lemon mixture in it with me to work along with 2 or 3 little water bottles for easy access while I was at work. Everyone kept asking me what I was doing and why, so I purchased a few more yellow books and passed them out.

The first three days I was miserable. I thought I was starving to death and that I was so hungry (even though I wasn't), it was all psychological, wanted to drink coffee and eat burritos so bad. I was angry at all the stupid people at the gym who were encouraging me to keep going. I got a few headaches throughout the day. I ended up taking walks during lunch when people were heating up their lunches in the office. I had to pee every 30 minutes to an hour, which I felt was helping cleaning me out.

Then after the third day, I felt skinny and light. I gained back all my energy, and I wasn't so grumpy. I decided to go to the gym and wok out lightly since I had energy. By the 10th day, I lost10 lbs, my nails were growing like crazy and I felt like I could leap 10 feet off the ground. (ok maybe not that high be I felt like a superhero). I also did a colonic the 10th day which put the icing on the cake. I felt squeaky clean inside, I had endless energy, and my water retention was gone, and fat shredded my body.

I was amazed by how I felt, and I did the master cleanse 5 more times the next following years. I actually enjoyed the lemonade mixture. I felt I broke the psychological barriers and cleansed my body of all the junk that accumulated in it.

K.K.

RESET CHALLENGE #8: THE MASTER CLEANSE

www.resetyourbody.com/wp-content/uploads/2013/02/The-Master-Cleanse-Daily-Routine.pdf

Join my Cleanse Support Group on Facebook now! Ask questions & interact. Don't do it alone!

www.ResetYourBody.com/SupportGroup

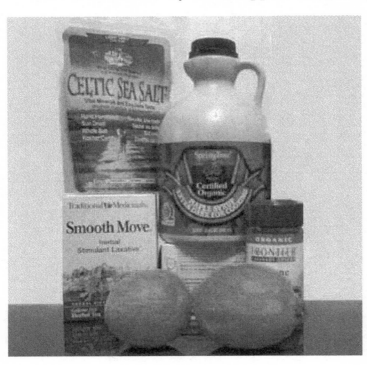

Overview:

- 10 days of actual fasting (5 days for first timers)
- +1 day to ease into the cleanse (optional)
- +2-3 days to ease out of the detox
- Total of 13-14 days
- Try to find someone to do the detox with you. The support is AWESOME!
- You will have lots of energy
- You will temporarily lose weight. But this is NOT a weight-loss diet!
- DRINK LOTS OF WATER

Track Your Progress:

Your Start Date: _____

Start Weight: _____

Your End Date: _____

End Weight: _____

IMPORTANT!! If you quit before the end, **DO NOT** just start eating normally right away. You MUST ease in to normal eating or you WILL get sick. Your body needs one to two days to rebuild the enzymes lost from not eating before you eat a burger or junk food. See the Ease Out days (raw fruits and veggies and soups).

2 days before the Master Cleanse

- Go shopping for your supplies

I recommend going to Trader Joes first for the lemons & larger maple syrup bottles and THEN go to a health food store to get whatever you couldn't find there.

INGREDIENTS

(If you have access to organic, it is far better to use it. But if you don't, then just use what you have.)

- 8 Gallons of pure distilled water
- 100 oz. GRADE B organic maple syrup (GRADE B has to be on the label)
- 1 small container of cayenne pepper
- 18 organic lemons (these will last three days; don't buy more yet or they will rot)
- Sea salt (FYI – pure sea salt is NOT WHITE. It looks pinkish or brownish)
- Any brand of laxative tea
- Any brand of herbal tea
- Optional: Oxygen-based intestinal cleanser pills (alternative to salt flush). Google "Mag07" or "OxyFlush."

1 day before (Ease in day)

- Eat only fruits and vegetables all day today
- Drink ten glasses of water today (fill up a jug if that will help you track it)
- Drink a serving of laxative tea before bed. (Stock up on these. You will get tired of the taste of lemonade.)

DAY 1

1. Salt flush – first thing in the morning, mix 1 tablespoon of sea salt with 1 quart of lukewarm water. Drink as quickly as possible. **Don't leave home for an hour. Trust me.**
2. Mix a full day's supply of lemonade (100 oz. daily serving):
   a. 100 oz. water
   b. 1 1/4 cup lemon juice
   c. 1 1/4 cup maple syrup (more or less to taste)
   d. 1 teaspoon cayenne pepper (more or less to taste)

3. Keep some with you at all times and leave some in the refrigerator for later.

4. DRINK LOTS OF WATER or HERBAL TEA THROUGHOUT THE DAY – wash out the toxins!

Alternate: Glass of lemonade then glass of water. If you are lightheaded or hungry or anything, drink more water. It will pass.

1. Drink a serving of laxative tea before bed.

 DAY 2 – DAY 10 (DAY 5 for first timers)

(You will notice that you end up drinking more water than lemonade each day)

1. Salt flush first thing in the morning
2. Mix a full day's supply of lemonade
3. Keep some with you at all times and leave some in the refrigerator for later.
4. DRINK LOTS OF WATER or HERBAL TEA THROUGHOUT THE DAY
5. Drink a serving of laxative tea before bed.

 DAY 11 (Ease out day 1)

1. Drink several glasses of orange juice or any fresh veggie or fruit juice (FRESH!)
2. DRINK LOTS OF WATER or HERBAL TEA THROUGHOUT THE DAY

 DAY 12 (Ease out day 2)

(Take more days if you have a weak stomach)

1. Drink several glasses of orange juice or any fresh veggie or fruit juice (FRESH!)
2. DRINK LOTS OF WATER or HERBAL TEA THROUGHOUT THE DAY
3. Raw fruit for lunch

4. Fruit or vegetable salad for dinner

 DAY 13

1. Normal eating may be resumed!

CONGRATULATIONS!! You are now Reset.

AFTER

IMPORTANT! You'll want to replace any good, beneficial bacteria lost as a side effect of the salt flushes. Keeps you from getting stomachaches and diarrhea, etc. Add one or any or all of these to your diet for the next week:

- Yogurt (with live cultures listed on the label)
- Kefir
- Sour cream
- Sauerkraut
- Pickles
- Probiotic supplements (any health store or online)

Don'ts and Extras

This is not required reading! If you are tired of reading and understanding this thing then STOP reading and get your butt busy...BUT some of you want more details, information, tricks, and extras (like me). This is for you!

Join my Cleanse Support Group on Facebook now! Ask questions & interact. Don't do it alone!

www.ResetYourBody.com/SupportGroup/

Low Blood Sugar folks & Diabetics – Two options

1. Substitute blackstrap molasses for the maple syrup
2. Stick to the Juice Cleanse for now. We need to keep you from passing the heck out!

Working out - Lots of people continue to work out while fasting. You will have enough energy to do some light exercise. With that said, I choose to not exercise while fasting:

1. I don't want to make myself hungry
2. We have a finite amount of energy. Why use it to build muscle for those ten days when I could have that energy to go towards cleaning up instead?
3. If I'm going to take ten days off from eating normally, I want the maximum benefits from it, so I let the cleaning process take precedence.

If the salt flush doesn't work (alternatives/adjustments)

- Lemon in water makes it easier to swallow and improves taste.
- Warm water is easier too.
- Psyllium husk is an expanding colon cleanser that basically bulks up and scours the inside of your colon. Only do this if you are NOT backed up. You need to have a flowing digestion already. You can alternate every other day – salt flush one day then psyllium husks the next (mornings).

If after three days the salt flush isn't working, that means you have a blockage somewhere. Stop the salt flush and take oxygen-based colon cleanser pills for the rest of the detox (NOT herbal colon cleansers – OXYGEN-BASED colon cleansing pills [(my favorites – Mag07 brand or OxyFlush brand]). Follow the instructions on the bottle

Speeding up the process – Speed up the body's attempts to flush out and remove toxins with profuse sweating daily (hot yoga, yoga, very hot bath for 20 minutes with Epsom/bath salts, 15-20 minutes in hot sauna and or steam room). Stay hydrated!

- **Using your mind to deepen the detox** – After day three, your body goes into autophagy mode…it scavenges itself for food, beginning with trash (fat, toxins, crystals, cysts, etc.).
- Envision those cells as tiny soldiers scouring the body and dissolving all the old bad rubbish that has built up over the years!

Headaches/pain/flu/fever – If you experience these, it most likely means you need to drink a lot more water. Ladies, a half gallon of water a day, at least. Guys, one gallon of water a day, at least. This is in addition to your lemonade. Your toxins are all stirred up but not getting out.

- It's normal to feel these for a half day or so. It will pass.
- If you have a lot of toxins to remove, it might take a few days of this…DON'T GIVE UP. Your body isn't in pain because of lack of food. It's in pain because of released toxins. If you don't let them flush out, they will just resettle back in and continue weakening your body!
- One day of lemonade only – don't make multiple days of lemonade. The enzymes in the lemons start to die pretty quickly after juicing them. One day at a time is enough.

Observe your body – IMPORTANT: Take inventory of your body! This might not apply until after the detox is completed and you are eating normally again.

- Skin, hair, nails, joints, breath, eyesight, etc. These things are not random. Keep track of what you notice about everything about your body. That is a sign that something was affected!

- **Takes more than 10 days of detoxing to remove 20–50+ years of buildup.**– Every time you detox, your body will target where it sees the most need. Let your body decide what to work on next. It might take three, four, five, six, or more detoxes for your body to get to the thing that you want Reset (it took me four).

- **No TV** – All the food commercials will kill you. Do yourself a favor – get a book or just watch movies!

Go back in time through the Cleanse Support Group on FB

www.facebook.com/groups/CleanseSupportGroup

Hundreds of people and pages of comments and suggestions and stories and tips and issues and highlights and lowlights from past detoxes.

Effects come AFTER the detox – While you are detoxing don't expect to see major positive changes in your body. It's like when you clean your house. Furniture is a mess, it smells like bleach. Dust is in the air. But after you're done cleaning (start to eat normally again) all the cleaned-up body systems process the nutrients better and then THEN –one to two weeks after the detox – you will notice the results. Take note!

Herbal tea – It is approved during this detox. After two to three days, your taste buds will be SUPER bored. Keep yourself strong! Have tasty herbal teas handy or grab one at a coffee shop. Flavor is your friend!

Your taste buds will reset – After a fast, your taste buds will no longer need overstimulation (sugars, artificial flavorings, etc.). You will have fewer cravings for "bad" processed foods!

If you cheat, don't quit! – You WILL have a moment of weakness. Don't just stop the detox if you do. One snack does not derail the massive benefits of your full body detox. Wipe your mouth. Tell the support group. And get back to the plan. Your body is too damn strong to let a cheat stop you! If you can't control your stomach for ten days, then who is really in charge here??

About Reset Challenge #8: The Master Cleanse

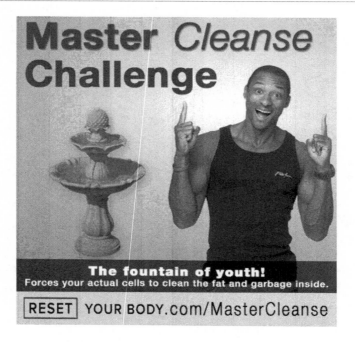

Welcome to the final Reset Challenge. You have arrived! This is the ultimate Reset Challenge and the most difficult and rewarding of the cleanses that I recommend.

The Master Cleanse is a safe, controlled, hypereffective method to remove years of toxic residue and impacted fecal matter and switch your body into an almost magic mode where your trillions and trillions of cells combine, at a microscopic level, to attack, devour, and eject foreign matter, fat, toxins, and garbage accumulated during your lifetime. This cleanse, in my opinion, is the one that turns back the hands of time to reverse aging and prolong your body's youth. (Pretty dramatic build up, huh?)

A Little history

Stanley Burroughs published the Master Cleanse back in the 1940s. I highly encourage you to read his short 62-page *The Master Cleanser*. It describes in detail how and why this is such a powerful health-promoting and almost eerily effective disease-eliminating method. Literally hundreds of thousands of people have benefited from this cleanse in the past 70 years, thanks to his book.

Criticisms

Chances are, you've either heard of someone or know someone that has tried the Master Cleanse and they either only made it a day or two OR they "got sick" doing it. Well in that case, "Why in the heck would I be fool enough to try this thing?? It's taking people out!" Well, hold on there, young buck!

As a matter of fact, I looked up Stanley Burroughs and the Master Cleanse on Wikipedia and most of the article was critical of the Master Cleanse:

"Nutritionist Jane Clark points to a lack of essential nutrients in this program, citing a deficiency of protein, vitamins, and minerals. As a result of these deficiencies, including far fewer calories than the recommended amount for health and optimum functioning, individuals on the diet may experience headaches and a variety of other symptoms in the short term and the diet is potentially harmful over the long term. The program has been described as an extreme fad or crash diet, and any weight lost during the fast can be expected to be regained once the diet is stopped. Dietician Keri Glassman has said those following the diet are 'guaranteed' to gain weight after stopping"

Tip #1 – When you search online for alternative/natural/or non-medical based health information, BE PREPARED FOR NEGATIVE INFORMATION. It's not the mainstream solution. So OF COURSE that means the masses do NOT believe in or subscribe to it (the definition of not being mainstream, right?) There should be ZERO surprise that MOST of the information about it will be negative. This is where you get to exercise your freedom of choice. No one article or book or speech is EVER allowed to form your entire opinion about something (health or any other topic). As a responsible adult, you must investigate multiple sources of information, consider these sources, and most important, use your common sense.

NOTE: The US Food and Drug Administration enforces the law that states, "only a drug can legally claim to treat, cure, or diagnose any disease."

We know that the disease, scurvy, is a vitamin C deficiency, and since the 1700s, sailors have intentionally brought lime juice during voyages to prevent scurvy. But limes are NOT a drug and so can't be called a cure. Now think about how this is a major problem now that obesity has recently be recognized as a disease.

Tip #2 – Get used to the idea that human behavior and success tends to occur on a bell curve (the VAST majority of people do the same things and experience average results. There will always be a small percentage that does something that gives them substandard results and there will be another small percentage that does something that gives them superior results – the outliers, as Malcolm Gladwell would put it).

Why am I talking about algebra all of a sudden? Well think about it. Football. How do most people in America perform on a scale of one to ten at playing football (one being Pop Warner 4-year-olds scrambling around randomly hitting one another regardless of ball possession and ten being NFL multi-million dollar contract players)? Most are between three and seven in skill level. Then there are a few of the super sucky. Then there are a few of the world-renowned variety. Thus is true in everything: career success, relationship success, income, happiness, health, etc.

So with that said, your job is to identify what the small percentage of the most successful people on the healthy bell curve are doing to achieve their stellar results, right? You, of course, know that the behaviors and beliefs of that super small group of the healthy elite (so to speak) will be things that the vast majority, the masses, are not at all doing (or they would have the same results).

Get used to being different. Get used to believing differently. Get used to not being fully understood by the masses. If you want have what the masses have, keep doing what the masses are doing.

What's the point? Someone is going to try to talk you out of this. Someone that cares about you and someone that you trust. They don't mean you any harm. I promise you, in the beginning, someone has tried to talk every successful person out of what made them a success (business, health…). Why? Because you are becoming an outlier, and those close to you don't want you to be different. They think they are protecting you. You just need to know where you stand BEFORE they come for you.

Summary of the day:

1. Salt flush to clean out slow-moving or stalled food in your 30 feet of intestines
2. Chug water like mad all day to flush out toxins
3. Drink up to one gallon of lemonade drink
4. No solid food
5. Laxative tea before bed

Behind the Scenes:

See previous chapter about salt flush.

Let your cells do all the work

The entire purpose of the fasting and Master Cleanses and even Water Fasting (that's water ONLY and nothing else – even I'm too scared to try that one), is to put your body in a controlled state of hunger so that your cells begin to scavenge your body to remove the garbage. That's pretty much it. Your body knows where it needs to focus first. Your body knows how to do it. We just need to flip the switch that starts the whole process. And how, pray tell, do we do that? We stop stuffing out faces nonstop all day long.

Imagine that you are back in caveman times. In case you forgot, we, as a species, have spent more time as cavemen and hunters and gatherers, than we have living in cities. So close your eyes and follow along here.

There you are, waking up in your cave (because the sun is shining on your face). What's the first thing you do? Reach for an

Eggo waffle and pop it in the toaster and get started on a cup of hot coffee? Not so much. You wake up wondering where your next meal is going to come from. You wander outside, eating some berries and mushrooms along the way. You meet up with Grog and Ugh and Mog, and you all start the daily task of looking for something big and muscular that will provide a nice high-energy meal for the group. Maybe you find some unlucky animal that day, maybe you don't. This is your everyday existence. Think about being in the woods, without technology to help you as a hunter. The odds aren't in your favor every day. Here's what you DON'T do. You DON'T spend all day long with an endless parade of foodstuffs flowing from your dirty little hands into your mouth. You are mildly hungry the vast majority of the time. (Don't worry, you're not suffering. You're used to this. It's just a part of life. No cavemen were harmed in the making of this flashback).

So what does a human body do when it's not expending energy performing the number one energy-consuming task of digesting food? It uses all of that energy and all of those resources to heal and repair itself. As we all know, doing a little bit every day prevents build up and prevents us from having to do a LOT someday. (Ask any bachelor how this philosophy applies to cleaning his flat). Fortunately, our caveman ancestors' bodies had ample opportunity most days, and certainly most weeks, to take advantage of the body's clean-up mode to remove toxic, fat, garbage load. But we 21st century cavemen, with our constant supply of food (very taxing on the energy scale) and our super heavy toxic load, we can literally go an entire lifetime and NEVER have our body switch into clean-up mode. AMAZING if you think about it. Something that happened to our ancestors, almost daily, may NEVER happen to us. (On the flip side, you get to play with an iPhone every day, but cousin Grog has never had the pleasure of asking Siri to "Find Chinese food near me." That cave dude missed out).

Laxative Tea

One of the most noticeable effects from these the final three Challenges will be the cleaning out of old impacted fecal matter from your gut. I know. It's nasty to think about that. But the only thing more nasty than thinking about years old food, rotting and cooking at 98 degrees in a dark, moist area (aka your intestines) is the disgusting effect that they've been having on your surrounding organs AND the less-than-flower-fresh emissions that are slowing seeping from the top of that tube (your mouth) and the bottom of that tube (your bum).

Got the visual yet?

The laxative tea helps accelerate the removal of that from your body. You take the tea at night and its job is to loosen up years of impacted food, like Drano down a clogged sink. Some of that food has been in there so long, and it's so dried out, it is literally as hard as a rock, and it will take continuous attempts to loosen it up and break it free. Be patient. In the morning, you do the salt flush and it pushes out anything that was loosened up. And you repeat the cycle each day during the cleanse. Depending on how much you had in you, you'll notice some pretty darn significant slimming of your waist.

The Ingredients: So what's doing what here?

Maple Syrup – Grade B maple syrup, not to be confused with the lighter shades and other grades of maple syrup, has the most mineral content of all of the grades. It provides your body with the calories and energy needed to keep active and alert all day. Do not use honey or any other substitutes for Grade B maple syrup UNLESS you have lower blood sugar or you are diabetic. In that case, you need something with more sugar content. Blackstrap molasses is your substitute. (You may add less syrup if you are overweight, or you may add more syrup if you are underweight.)

Lemon – Ancient Egyptians believed that eating lemons was an effective protection against poisons. Lemons are a strong antibacterial and antiviral, and an immune buster. And even though lemons are an acid fruit, they become alkaline as they are digested and assimilated. What the heck does that mean? When your body is sick, it becomes acidic, so consuming alkaline substances helps to counteract that acidity to bring you back to a healthy state. Think of it like using Tums or an antacid to neutralize heartburn (stomach acid).

Cayenne Pepper – Cayenne pepper breaks up mucus in your body. Mucus is used by your body to trap and hold toxins so they don't flow freely around your body causing damage. It's like fly paper. You know how your nose starts to run when you eat some super spicy food? That's what we're trying to do here: get the mucus that's holding all those toxins flowing so that your body can sneeze, cough, and drip it out of you. Let it flow!

Master Cleanse vs. Juice Cleanse

One question that I get quite often is "What's better? The Juice Cleanse or the Master Cleanse?" Well it's not really about which is "better" because they are very different processes.

The Juice Cleanse is designed to super saturate your 100 trillion cells with a nutrient overload and feed the undernourished cells to make up for years and years of an inefficient diet and poor eating choices and to supercharge cancerous and dying organs and body parts (remember the "water the brown grass analogy"). Juicing is doing just that. It's like sprinkling the best fertilizer and watering your dead and dying lawn. Give it all the food that it needs deep, deep down.

The Master Cleanse is kind of the opposite. It's designed to put the body into that controlled state of hunger (temporarily) so that your cells begin to scavenge the body for nutrients. It dissolves and devours those years of excess fat cells and crystal deposits and cysts and tumors and toxic deposits and scar tissue and cellulite - ANYTHING that isn't essential to your body's functioning. Think of it as setting loose a few billion Pacmen in your body, all hell-bent on eating garbage! This is why I choose to do the Master Cleanse every year. I want the cleanup. (Obviously, when you juice, your body will do some scavenging and clean up at the cellular level as well. Just not to the extent and depth of the Master Cleanse.)

The Perfect Mix

So what would be a great way to maximize juicing and the Master Cleanse? Do both! Let your body clean out any garbage that has collected. Do a five to ten day Master Cleanse. Then super charge your body's cells every day or week by adding a few glasses of fresh juice to your diet every day or every week. It's similar to taking care of a garden. You water and feed your crop every day then every so often, you pull weeds and remove the pests.

How Often?

Your goal will really dictate how often you Master Cleanse. If you have a deep, persistent, chronic disease or illness, or you are obese and you have an excess of fat, you may decide to do 10 days or more (up to 40 days according to Stanley Burroughs) three to four times per year, with at least 30 days between each to give your body time to rebuild and repair. As always, LISTEN TO YOUR BODY.

Replenish any lost beneficial gut bacteria

One side effect of the salt flush (power washing your insides) is not only does it flush out old food, toxins, and waste, it also washes out billions of the good bacteria. A healthy person has billions of bacteria in their intestines that aid in digestion and break down and assimilate foods and nutrients. If we aren't careful, after a few salt flushes, once we go back to eating, we can have digestive issues for a while: stomach pains after eating, diarrhea, and general stomach discomfort.

The way around that is to accelerate the replacement of the good guys.

- Eating fermented and cultured foods (yogurts, sauerkraut, pickles, kefir, etc.)
- Taking powerful probiotic supplements (1 billion plus live organisms – I know if sounds like you're putting a gaggle of alien monsters in your mouth. Don't freak out!)

- Focus on increasing these in your diet for one to two days right at the completion of your Juice Cleanse.

LIVER CLEANSE & GALL BLADDER FLUSH

Taken from (more details):

curezone.com/cleanse/liver/huldas_recipe.asp

Join my Cleanse Support Group on Facebook now! Ask questions & interact. Don't do it alone!

www.ResetYourBody.com/SupportGroup

Purpose:

-Cause the liver and gallbladder to eject "gallstones," thus clearing blocked liver bile ducts

Overview:

- Print instructions and *READ ENTIRELY TWICE*
- Twenty hours long (2 p.m. on Day1 till around 10 a.m. on Day 2)

1. Epsom salt dilates bile ducts and cleans colon
2. Olive oil causes liver to spasm and squeeze out hardened deposits
3. Grapefruit juice speeds up process and encourages gallbladder spasms
4. Epsom salt washes stones out

Things to Expect:

- 20-70 small green stones
- There is no pain passing stones
- If you have no stones the first time, don't worry. Repeat in 1-2 weeks

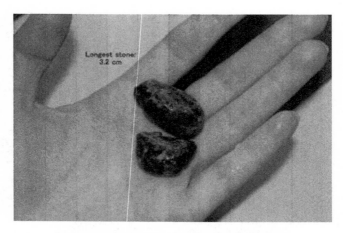

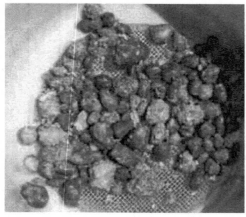

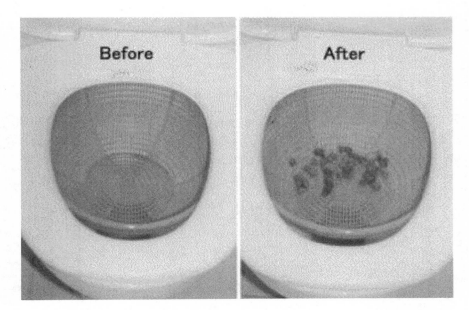

Before **After**

Recommended: You can substitute the three cups of water that is used in this recipe to dissolve Epsom salt with three cups freshly pressed grapefruit juice or freshly pressed apple juice. That way you will not notice the unpleasant taste of Epsom salt.

- Ornithine capsules
- 3 cups water

Choose a day like Friday or Saturday for the cleanse, since you will be able to rest the next day until around 10 a.m.

- Take no medicines, vitamins, or pills that you can do without; they could prevent success.
- Eat a no-fat breakfast and lunch such as cooked cereal with fruit, fruit juice, bread and preserves or honey (no butter or milk), baked potato or other vegetables with salt only. This allows the bile to build up and develop pressure in the liver. Higher pressure pushes out more stones.

2 p.m. Do not eat or drink (other than water) after 2 p.m. If you break this rule, you could feel quite ill later. Get your Epsom salts ready. Mix 4 tablespoons in 3 cups water and pour this into a jar. This makes four servings, 3/4 (three fourths) cup each. Set the jar in the refrigerator to get ice cold (this is for convenience and taste only).

6 p.m. Drink one serving (3/4 cup) of the ice-cold Epsom salts. If you did not prepare this ahead of time, mix 1 tablespoon in 3/4 cup water now. You may add 1/8 teaspoon vitamin C powder to improve the taste. You may also drink a few mouthfuls of water afterwards or rinse your mouth. Get the olive oil and grapefruit out to warm up.

8 p.m. Repeat by drinking another 3/4 cup of Epsom salts. You haven't eaten since 2 p.m. but you won't feel hungry. Get your bedtime chores done. The timing is critical for success.

9:45 p.m. Pour 1/2 cup (measured) olive oil into the pint jar. Wash grapefruit twice in hot water and dry; squeeze by hand into the measuring cup. Remove pulp with fork. You should have at least 1/2 cup, more (up to 3/4 cup) is best. You may use part lemonade. Add this to the olive oil. Also, add 1 dropper full of Black Walnut Tincture. Close the jar tightly with the lid and shake hard until watery.

Now visit the bathroom one or more time, even if it makes you late for your 10 p.m. drink. Don't be more than 15 minutes late. You will get fewer stones.

10 p.m. Drink the potion you have mixed. Take four ornithine capsules with the first sips to make sure you will sleep through the night. Take eight if you already suffer from insomnia. Drinking through a large plastic straw helps it go down more easily. You may use oil and vinegar salad dressing or straight honey to chase it down between sips. Have these ready in a tablespoon on the kitchen counter. Take it all to your bedside if you want, but drink it standing up. Get it down within five minutes (fifteen minutes for very elderly or weak persons).

Lie down immediately. Lie on right side. You might fail to get stones out if you don't. The sooner you lie down the more stones you will get out. Be ready for bed ahead of time. Don't clean up the kitchen. As soon as the drink is down, walk to your bed and **lie on right side** with your head up high on the pillow. Try to think about what is happening in the liver. Try to keep perfectly still for at least 20 minutes. You may feel a train of stones traveling along the bile ducts like marbles. There is no pain because the bile duct valves are open (thank you Epsom salts). Go to sleep. You may fail to get stones out if you don't.

Next morning. Upon awakening, take your third dose of Epsom salts. If you have indigestion or nausea wait until it is gone before drinking the Epsom salts. You may go back to bed. Don't take this potion before 6 a.m.

This is about when you'll start passing stones!

Two Hours Later. Take your fourth (the last) dose of Epsom salts. You may go back to bed again.

OR...This is when you'll start passing stones!

After Two More Hours you may eat. Start with fruit juice. Half an hour later, eat fruit. One hour later, you may eat regular food but keep it light. By supper, you should feel recovered.

How well did you do?

Expect diarrhea in the morning.

FYI – I had ZERO stones my first time. But I could feel that something was going on in there. So I did it two weeks later. Voila. I've eliminated 50-70 stones every time since.

Join my Cleanse Support Group on Facebook now! Ask questions & interact. Don't do it alone!

www.ResetYourBody.com/SupportGroup

About the Liver Cleanse

It's kind of an interesting story how I came across this cleanse. I met a man that had been in the World Trade Center on 9/11. I met him seven years after the fact, and he was still plagued by health issues that resulted from that day. Do you remember seeing the footage as the buildings collapsed? Huge clouds of smoke and dust and debris. The air was filled with soot and who knows what. Everyone that was there had to breath in that mess. Imagine breathing that in for a few minutes. So my friend had respiratory issues. Allergy issues. His body and his blood were just filled with tons of airborne toxic waste. So he told me about this liver cleanse that made him "feel like a brand new person" after he did it.

How clogged or damaged is your liver RIGHT NOW?

Test:

- Do you drink more than one spirit alcoholic beverage per day? (Vodka, tequila, rum, whiskey, etc.)
- Have you noticed that you have intense hangovers now but you didn't years ago?
- Does it take a long time to recover after heavy drinking the day before?
- Do you have brown spots on your skin?
- Does your body not process and break down fats very well?
- Has it been more than six months since your last liver detox?

No to all questions = PASS

Yes to any of those questions = FAIL. You may have a sluggish, clogged liver.

Your liver is constantly filtering and cleaning your blood 24 hours a day, 7 days a week, 365 days a year. For years and years and years. The more difficult we make that job with too much fat consumption and too many days of repeated alcohol consumption, the more clogged and damaged and overworked the liver gets.

These are the stones that build up in the liver and gallbladder of an otherwise healthy 20-30 year old. Disgusting, right? Hard to look at, right? Well, too late, if you failed the test above; they are most likely already in you.

We're not talking about a couple of these. Many people will pass 40, 50, 60, 70+ of these small stones after detoxing and flushing their liver.

You have two options:

1. Keep the stones in your liver and gallbladder; or
2. Do something to get them out so that your liver to returns to normal function.

What's going on?

Among other things, your liver creates bile. Bile is the greenish liquid that helps break down fats. So the liver has many bile ducts, tubes that squirt the bile into the gallbladder.

Over years of abuse, these bile ducts get clogged and deposits start to slow down the flow of bile. Basically a blockage in the tube.

Unclog the tubes

The purpose of the Liver Cleanse is to help your body naturally (without drugs and medication) remove that blockages quickly and safely so that you can have a stronger, more efficient liver.

How does the process work?

It literally takes less than one day: 20 hours
Start at 2 p.m. on Day 1 and you're done and back to normal by 10 a.m. on Day 2.

- **Step 1)** Choose a day. Pick a Friday or Saturday so that you have the following day until 10 a.m. at home
- **Step 2)** Stop eating at 2 p.m. on Day 1. We need a clear digestive tract so the ejected stones have a way out.
- **Step 3)** Drink 3/4 cup of special Epsom Drink at 6 p.m.
- **Step 4)** Drink 3/4 cup of special Epsom Drink at 8 p.m.
- **Step 5)** Drink 1 cup of special Liver Flush Drink at 10 p.m.
- **Step 6)** Go to bed
- **Step 7)** Drink 3/4 cup of special Epsom Drink when you wake in the morning (at this point you may start passing stones)
- **Step 8)** Drink 3/4 cup of special Epsom Drink two hours later (at this point you may start passing stones)
- **Step 9)** Two hours after that – YOU'RE ALL DONE and you have a new, more powerful liver.

Is it Safe?

YES! An emphatic yes! What's NOT safe is resorting to drugs and medications to try and mask the symptoms of a sluggish, damaged liver until one day your liver gives out on you.

The only things in the drinks are Epsom salts, olive oil, grapefruit juice, and apple juice, all in the right proportion and all with a purpose.

Your body

How your body reacts is unique. Drinking a high volume of water will help improve your results and will help to minimize any cleansing reactions. Many people (including me) do not pass stones on their first liver flush. Don't worry. Repeat it in two weeks and see the magic happen then. Some livers are more stubborn than others.

What about an herbal liver cleanse or liver cleanse teas?

Those are great solutions as well. But just like anything else, there are slower, more gradual ways to do things and there are more effective, deeper, accelerated ways to do things. You can choose what you think your body needs right now.

CLEANSE FREQUENTLY ASKED QUESTIONS (FAQs)

Q: "How many days should I cleanse for?"

A: First timers can do five days. Everyone else should shoot for ten days. You can certainly go longer. Read *The Master Cleanser* by Stanley Burroughs for details.

Q: "How often should I cleanse?"

A: I recommend you take a month between cleanses. Let your body build up between cleansings. I cleanse once per year now. If you need to be more aggressive (excess fat, major health issues, thrill seeker) you can cleanse as often as you like.

Q: "How many times have you cleansed?"

As of 2014: I have cleansed thirteen times. My first cleanse was a 10-day master cleanse in 2007 (I do that once a year). My first liver flush cleanse was 2009 (I do that twice a year). I've done the Veggie Cleanse twice. I've done the Juice Cleanse once. I do a 1-Day Reset (mini Veggie Cleanse) every few months when I need to kick-start things.

Q: "I have a cold/flu now. Should I wait to start my cleanse?"

A: Actually, starting a cleanse will absolutely help you heal faster. Flooding your body with live enzymes, not expending energy digesting food, letting your body go into garbage-scavenge mode is EXACTLY what you want to do right away. Stay the plan.

Q: "Do the ease in and ease out days count as cleanse days?"

A: No, they don't. So a 10-day cleanse is 10 days of cleansing. Easing in or out are extra days to count.

Q: "What if I do it wrong?"

A: Don't worry! It's not about perfection. Just do your best. Be sure to read the instructions THOROUGHLY two to three times BEFORE you start.

Q: "What's the minimum number of days I can do?"

A: Three days. The longer you go at a time, the better. (e.g., A 10-day cleanse is far more effective than two 5-day cleanses spread apart.)

Q: "What's the maximum amount of days?"

A: Veggie Cleanse – no limit. Juice Cleanse – 40 days is all I'm comfortable recommending. Master Cleanse – 40 days per *The Master Cleanser* Book. NOTE: After 10 days, salt flush twice weekly. After three weeks, salt flush once per week.

Q: "Do I need to read the original *The Master Cleanser* book by Stanley Burroughs?"

A: No, you don't. But I have found that everyone that has read it has completed their full cleanse (hint).

Q: "I can't find a good time to cleanse. Now what?"

A: You always have a choice. If your job has you too busy, you are choosing that job over your health. If you are travelling too much, you are choosing those trips over your health. If you are afraid, you are choosing fear over growth. You always have a choice.

Q: "What do I say if people say I'll lose too much weight?"

A: Tell them you are not doing this to lose weight. Tell them you are doing this to remove years of toxic waste from your body (even possible pre-cancerous cells). Some of that is in the weight you've lost. You will regain your body's normal, healthy weight right after the cleanse.

Q: "What do I say if people say this is stupid?"

A: Remind yourself to not be 1 one of the 19. (Five percent of people get what they want out of life. That's 1 out of 20.)

Q: "How do I find the schedule of group cleanses?"

A: First Monday = 1-Day Reset. Second Monday = Veggie Cleanse. Third Monday = Juice Cleanse. Fourth Monday = Master Cleanse. Join my Facebook Reset Cleanse Support Group @ www.facebook.com/groups/CleanseSupportGroup

Q: "What if I didn't lose weight on my cleanse?"

A: That means one of three things: 1) you did not do the daily salt flush to wash out intestinal waste; 2) the toxins and waste your body removed (pre-cancer cells, cysts, crystals, scar tissue, wrinkles, etc.) didn't weigh much; or 3) you probably lost INCHES and didn't track it (if you are overweight, measuring your arms and waist and legs would have been a better indicator of body changes).

Q: "What can I do if I travel all the time?"

A: Two options: 1) Cancel your travel plans for ten days (recommended), or 2) do the Veggie Cleanse and the Juice Cleanse on the road (buying juices or vegetarian dishes).

Q: "I don't feel any side effects during my cleanse. Is it working?"

A: So you haven't eaten any solid food in days or you have been flooding your body with billions of live vegetable enzymes and fiber. YES, IT'S WORKING! Just because you aren't having headaches or pains or discomfort doesn't mean pre-cancerous cells aren't being removed, weak organs aren't being repaired, etc. Trust me. Don't wish for uncomfortable side effects as proof.

Q: "How do I convert quarts to ounces and teaspoons to tablespoons?"

A: The Internet!

Q: "Do I need to ease into the cleanse?"

A: No, you don't NEED to. I don't. Many don't. It's helpful if you eat a very processed, junk food diet right now, though.

Q: "What if I have low blood sugar issues?"

A: This is an important issue for the Juice Cleanse (Add more fruit juice if you feel light-headed) and the Master Cleanse (see the instructions on using blackstrap molasses instead of maple syrup).

Q: "What juicer do you recommend?"

A: Personally, I've had a Breville Juice Fountain Plus for eight years. It's easy to clean and strong enough to juice apples without preslicing them. ($150 at the time)

Q: "How many days do I have to cleanse to make it on the WALL of Winners?"

A: Just make it through how many days you committed to.

Q: "Where do I send my picture for the WALL of Winners?"

A: Email to me@terrygivens.com or post on the Reset Cleanse Support Page

Q: "How do I eat afterwards to keep the benefits of my cleanse?"

A: Stick to my 6 Rules to Eat By section. Chemical-free meat and plants, no breads or processed carbs.

Q: "Do I REALLY need to do the salt flush every day?"

A: YES. Without the salt flush you won't remove the old impacted gunk in your intestines that is making you sick and adding inches to your waist, and you won't remove the stirred-up toxins fast enough and you may feel more sick DURING the cleanse. Trust me, everyone hates the salt flush. Me too! But sometimes we do it because it's good for us.

Q: "Does it get easier every time?"

A: Absolutely. Every single time! Remember the first time tying your shoe? Or driving a car? Your body adjusts. You need less food to have the same energy.

Q: "What if I can't buy probiotic supplements?"

A: They are not REQUIRED. They simply help to speed up the replacement of good gut bacteria. See the list of cultured foods to eat, and they will do exactly what you need.

Q: "Do I have to use organic everything?"

A: NO. You are not REQUIRED to use anything organic. Personally, I will ALWAYS choose organic for the stronger medicinal qualities it provides my cleanse.

Q: "When should I quit trying?"

A: NEVER. EVER. QUIT! You do not fail until you stop trying.

Q: "This time is so much worse than my previous cleanses. What gives?"

A: GOOD! That means this time your body is choosing to cleanse something that is causing a different detox reaction in you. Interesting when your body chooses what to work on.

Q: "Is it normal to feel bloated?"

A: Yes. Most won't experience it, some will. It's temporary.

Q: "Is there a minimum amount of juice/lemonade to drink each day?"

A: No. As long as you keep your water intake very high (shoot for a gallon of water) then how much or how little juice or lemonade you drink is 100% up to you.

Q: "Squeezing lemons is killing my hands. Ideas?"

A: Buy a lemon squeezer at a store or online.

Q: "How long does the salt flush take?"

A: You need to chug it down as quickly as possible (five minutes or less). For some it will take 15 minutes to cause a movement, some will take 90 minutes or more. It can last, off and on, for 30-120 minutes. The more hydrated you are and the less clogged you are inside, the faster it will start and the shorter it will last. Drinking more water after your salt flush and staying on your feet will speed things up.

Q: "Can I work out during the cleanse?"

A: Yes. Many continue working out while cleansing. Others, like myself, choose not to. Read why in my cleanse instructions.

Q: "Can I take supplements during my cleanse?"

A: It's recommended that you do NOT take supplements and you discontinue any nonvital medications while cleansing. The cleanse is trying to force your body to adjust and repair itself and recalibrate your body to what a "normal" state of being is. Artificially modifying it with supplements and medications gives a false "normal" state.

Q: "Can I season my vegetables?"

A: YES! Think about what seasonings and spices are? Plants and roots and herbs – very natural! I use lots and lots of seasonings

Q: "Can I do oxygen colon cleansing pills instead of the salt flush?"

A: Only use oxygen colon cleansing pills if you have a medical reason or extreme discomfort from the salt flush. The pills are good, but they have nowhere near the "power washing" effect that the salt flush has.

Q: "Is herbal tea the same as laxative tea?"

A: No. Herbal tea refers to any tea made of natural herbs (plant parts) vs. artificially flavored and sweetened teas. Laxative tea is a tea that induces bowel movements.

Q: "Can I use a blender (Ninja, Vitamix, etc.) instead of a juicer for the Juice Cleanse?"

A: No. Juicers remove the fiber and pulp so that the liquid bypasses your body's digestive system. Blenders do not. (They are healthy and great, but they are not a replacement during a Juice Cleanse)

Have you heard the story about a truck that got stuck under a bridge? A box truck was attempting to pass under a large bridge. As the truck driver approached the structure, he felt there was enough room to clear the bottom of the steel and concrete deck of the bridge. But as he was passing under, he suddenly hear a loud screeching noise! The screech turned in to a grind and the lurching truck came to a dead stop! It was now locked under the bridge and could go neither forward or backward. Putting the transmission in reverse, or one of the forward gears was no use as the vehicle was now firmly lodged directly under the bridge. Traffic came to a complete standstill and, naturally, the local authorities were called out to examine the situation. How would they get the truck out from under the bridge? A tow truck was sent out to try to pull the vehicle free. A county engineer arrived to examine this difficult situation. There were deep discussions and many measurements were made. Various calculations were performed to determine how much of the truck or bridge would be destroyed if the vehicle was simply yanked or pulled out! If too much of the bridge's concrete was broken in the process, it might cause the bridge to become unsafe. What if road equipment was brought in to cut a grove into the road under the vehicle tires to lower it? What if heavy equipment was brought in to lift the bridge just a few inches? Traffic continued to back up and discussions raged on as frustrated workers and authorities pondered this difficult problem. A crowd also gathered around the scene to watch all the exciting activity and hubbub. Then something funny happened. A little boy who had previously been riding his bicycle and had stopped to glare said to the man, "Why not let the air out of the tires?" "What?" stated the worker in incredulous shock! "What did you say?" The boy repeated, "Why not let the air out of the tires?" From this simple observation and statement, an easy and effective solution was found to a difficult problem that had confounded some very bright and energetic people!

This reminds me of America's health care problems: misguided, complicated solutions for a lifestyle problem.

Hm.....IT'S TIME TO LET THE AIR OUT OF THE TIRES, MY FRIENDS.

Improving Results

There are always some people that get better results at the same things. Have you noticed that? Give two people the same task or the same challenge, and one of them just does it better than the next guy (the kid that blew the grading curve in school or the executive assistant that makes multitasking look natural). Well, guess what? The same is true with people that detox and cleanse their bodies. Good news is, after meeting hundreds of cleansers, I can give you the inside scoop on the secrets, tips and tricks, and systems that gave them the edge. READY?

- Schedule the time ASAP – There is never a good time to cleanse. Unless you live under a rock, there is never a magical five to ten days where you have nothing on your social calendar. Block the time off now.
- List out your whys – Write down a list of why you're doing this (things you want to change or prevent). List your specific goals (weight, energy, activities).
  Use daily mantras – Repeat an empowering health statement daily. For example, "I hold in me the power to build the body I deserve," or "I'm a healthy person. I always make the right decision," or, "There is nothing to fear. I am doing the right thing."
- Find a partner – Have someone else cleansing with you. Or join my Reset Cleanse Support group. Just don't do it alone!
- Envision – See in your mind's eye all the live enzymes in the vegetables and fruits dissolving and removing years of old food and waste. See in your mind's eye your cells as millions of tiny soldiers attacking and destroying toxins and bacteria and viruses in your body.

COLONICS

Your colon doesn't need any help eliminating waste matter when we do what we're supposed to do by eating a high fiber diet, drinking large amounts of water, avoiding too much processed food, and getting vigorous exercise. So if you fit that bill, you can totally skip this section because – GREAT NEWS – you don't need this AT ALL. Now, for the other 99% of us – LISTEN UP!

Pop Quiz! What's 30 feet long and elastic and starts at your mouth and ends are your butt? BINGO – your intestines (that word just sounds nasty, doesn't it?)

In regards to our bowels, Dr. Richard Schulze, an herbal expert, a medical doctor with 30 years experience, and a healer of literally thousands, says:

1. The one organ that could be creating the most problems and negatively effecting other organs, without a doubt, is the colon

   and

2. It must be cleared out and functional to ensure that any detox regime is beneficial. It's the way out of toxins

Close your eyes and envision what you think your organs look like inside your body. If you're like most you see a heart (shaped like a Valentine) over on the left side, then you see your stomach, your lungs down the ways a bit, then you see your kidneys kind of behind those somewhere, etc. all nice and spaced out, right?

The reality: It's tight and crowded and hot in there. Imagine shoulder-to-shoulder, standing room only in a crowded subway car in Japan with 98-degree humidity during rush hour with no air conditioning and everyone is wearing a bathing suit. That's what your insides look like. Everything is touching everything else. Slipping, sliding, rubbing. Any infections, problems, or ailments can easily be passed around the organs.

So as your colon expands to handle slow-moving, dry, impacted fecal matter that has been building up over time, it starts to CRUSH other organs to take up space. Crushed organs don't work as well (wink, wink). Quite often, diseases of one part of the body are really stemming from the crushing of neighboring organs by the bowels or by the slow leaking of toxic waste into your bloodstream.

Think about these possibilities:

- Crushed heart leads to palpitations or irregular heartbeat – you think it's your heart.
- Crushed lungs – you think you have asthma.
- Crushed uterus leads to painful, agonizing periods – your colon wraps around your uterus.
- Crushed prostate leads to prostate issues.
- What about crushed pancreas, crushed kidneys?

Years of backed up waste in your colon slowly start to leak into your bloodstream, slowly and steadily wreaking havoc in seemingly unrelated parts of the body…slowly and steadily…

How is it supposed to work?

When observing infants and tribal-based cultures we figure out that:

We should have two to three bowel movements each day, about 20 minutes after each meal.

What's the reality?

Americans have two to five BM's per week.

That's about 14 missed BMs per week, 58 missed BMs per month, 792 missed BMs per year!!! Where is the poo going???

FACT - In 2013, sixty thousand people died of colon cancer (more than prostate cancer and breast cancer) * American Cancer Society. Cancer Facts & Figures 2013. Atlanta: American Cancer Society; 2013

What's a colonic?

First off, it is NOT the same as a colonoscopy! A colonoscopy is a diagnostic procedure that is usually done after the age of 50 to screen for cancer and possible polyps. It involves drinking some pretty unpleasant chemicals to make way for a camera to enter the bowels.

A colonic, on the other hand, is really a way of life. It can be performed daily, weekly, monthly, or on a yearly basis.

DEFINITION: A colonic is the infusion of water into the rectum by a colon therapist to cleanse and flush out the colon. It is also called colonic hydrotherapy or colon irrigation.

Benefits of a colonic

- Makes digestive system more effective
- Maintains regularity and prevents constipation
- Increases energy
- Reduces allergies
- Reduces cravings
- Increases fertility
- Eliminates toxins leaking into your bloodstream
- FAST!

Yup...the tube in the butt! Trust me, as a man, I was not looking forward to something going IN my EXIT-only zone. I spent years rationalizing why I didn't need to do it, but in the end (no pun intended) testimonies, research, and common sense won over, and I can honestly say that I believe that EVERY HUMAN BEING needs to have this procedure done. The level of internal cleaning is unparalleled! I'm sold. Now I'm going to sell you.

I'm going to tell you a story.

In 2013, after finishing my annual 10-day Master Cleanse, I went to have a post-cleanse colonic. I had had three colonics before that – once a year for the previous three years. There are two types of colonics: Closed System and Open system. Those previous colonics were closed system colonics. You lay on the bed, the colonic therapist is there with you to insert the tube and assist with the process the entire time. They control the flow of water in and out of you, and when the technician releases the water, the waste from your colon flows out through the tube. Think drinking an ice cream shake using a straw. (Sorry for the nasty visual!)

But for THIS colonic, I decided to do an open system colonic. Instead of a person inserting the tube and staying with you the entire time, you basically do that on your own. You lay on a table with your legs up and a built-in "drain sewer" and you insert the much smaller open system tube yourself. The technician comes in a few times during the procedure to check on you and start and stop the water, etc., but you are mostly in private for this one.

I TOTALLY prefer the open system vs. the closed system!

1. No one else is looking at my butt and sticking tubes in and out of it!
2. I control the flow of water and waste in and out simply by barely tightening my anus and releasing it.
3. Larger, hardened waste could come out around the pencil-sized open system water tube vs. those larger, hardened wastes not being able to fit through the closed system tube. (That has happened to me.)

So the nice lady shows me into the room and tells me to take off my clothes, put on the hospital gown, lay on the table, lube up the tip, and stick it in the ole rump. After psyching myself up to do the thing that needed to be done (trust me, you almost do NOT feel tube; I wasn't sure it was even in initially), she comes back in, turns on the water, and tells me to lightly squeeze my anus as long as I can to seal the water and let it fill up my lower colon. Once I feel the need, I relax and the water – along with whatever loosened inside me – flows out and down a type of trough/sewer deal. Down alongside the bed, there is a clear viewing tube so that you can marvel at the nastiness at it leaves your body (proof that it's actually working!)

If you think about it, it's common sense. Let's say you cooked spaghetti one night. You mixed the sauce in with the noodles and let it sit in a pan overnight. The next day that stuff is all dried out and caked in there right? So the million-dollar question is what do you do to clean out that pot? BINGO! Run water into it and let it soak to loosen up the leftovers. It's the exact same thing with a colonic. You're just loosening up your own spaghetti.

…YEAH! (Nasty, but I bet you get the point!)

So there I am on the table. And mind you, I'm no newbie to cleaning out my gut. By this time I've had seven years of cleansing under my belt – Master Cleanses, Veggie Cleanses, and a couple of Liver Flushes a couple of time a year. I'd guess that I'd had over 40 salt flushes by then. (That stuff cleans you out!) I eat a very clean diet accompanied with tons of daily vegetables and fruits. I drink lots of water every day, and I have a narrow waist and athletic abs. (I'd date me!) BUT LET ME TELL YOU WHAT CAME OUT.

At first, there were these hard, round little balls. They came rolling down the viewing tube (you can lightly feel them as they pop out – NO PAIN). Then I'd held in for a bit and released, and I felt this tumbling of waste coming out. I could see it just flowing through the viewing tube. (It's yucky, but it's like watching a train wreck;, you can't look away!) I couldn't figure out where it was coming from! This went on for 45 minutes. At one point, I held in the water as long as I could then let go and sludge literally filled up the viewing tube for about ten seconds (the viewing tube was three inches wide) Where the hell did that come from?!?

I'm a guy that thinks that I'm pretty clean on the inside. Can you imagine what a person that lives a normal American lifestyle would have on their insides? What would come out of them for

45 minutes? What would come out of YOU for 45 minutes straight? All fears and jokes aside, you may have some old impacted food inside you slowing your digestion and crushing your other organs causing all types of seemingly nonrelated symptoms throughout your body. A colonic is the fastest way to expedite the removal of all that built up toxic load, so that you can get on to living for tomorrow, instead of having to constantly be dealing with yesterday's consequences.

You have to do something different if you want different results.

Difference between a colonic and an enema:

<u>Colonic:</u>	<u>Enema:</u>
• Cleanses the entire length of colon	• Cleanses lower colon only
• Multiple infusions of water	• Single fusion of water
• Must go to a facility	• Can be done at home
• Just show up	• Requires education on technique

Top belly flatteners you can do on your own

Obviously, you don't need to trek all the way to a colonic clinic as the only way to remove bowel waste and slim your waistline. Billions of humans have been able to do it without colonics throughout history. ALL of these will involve:

1. High levels of water consumption and
2. High levels of fiber intake (raw vegetables and fruits – the highest fiber of any food)

Here are seven things you can start doing TODAY, on your own, to effectively break up, dissolve, and safely remove pounds and pounds of years old sewage laying around in your bowels.

1. Vibrating belt

People ALWAYS laugh when I bring this up. Why is that so darn funny? Remember black-and-white video footage of a chubby guy standing on a machine attached to a long belt that would vibrate and cycle back and forth, jiggling his belly like mad? Think about how that might loosen that guy's dried up, stuck together "spaghetti" inside him. Shakes it and loosens it, huh? Gets it moving, huh? Do these things actually shake enough to do anything? HELL, YEAH! I've experimented with a few and a good high-powered one will shake the living crap out of you (pun intended). It had me sweating and tired after less than a minute! Use daily for as long as you feel. Start slow – five to ten minutes.

> TIPS: Many will say that it "burns fat." I'm pretty sure the actual manufacturers don't even know how the belts they are selling truly work. They don't "burn" but they do give your insides a good shaking to break up what's stuck in there.

2. Percussion massager

Beat it up! You can use this little number on your lower abdomen while you are lying on the couch or in bed. Start slowly. You may make yourself feel nauseous with all of the vibrating, so stop and take a break for a few minutes if that's the case. Move it around your abdomen. Envision what part of your colon you're massaging while you do it. Use daily for as long as you feel. Start slow: five to ten minutes.

TIP: Move it in a clock-wise rotation to go WITH the intestinal movement.

3. Abdominal massage

Lay on your back. Place your hands on your abdomen. Move them around to find sore and tender spots. Massage and press on these spots for 20 minutes, twice per day. What are you trying to do? The poor man's percussion massage! Loosen up and knead your gut to help your body remove the junk. You can use massage oil if you like, but it's not required.

> TIP: When you're proficient, do them while sitting and bend forward and press the abdomen hard in order to reach the deepest parts of your abdomen.

4. Herbal colon cleansers

These can be teas or pills or powders, etc. Unlike drug-based laxatives and colon cleansers, which cause unnatural side effects like weakening of your intestinal muscular function, herbal-based colon cleansers stimulate and activate and enhance your colon's natural function (instead of replacing it).

Dr. Schulze tells a story of a man in Hawaii that took 49 capsules of his highly powerful herbal colon cleanser. The bowel movements that finally started had him on the toilet for 24 hours. This man, a 400+ pound man, proceeded to lose 50 pounds of colon and intestinal crap! Yes, really!

There are countless colon cleansing kits at any local health food store or online. Don't be afraid to try different types (teas vs. pills, etc.) and try different brands. Find what your body reacts best to and continue with what works for you.

TIP: If you do use natural laxative and colon cleansing herbs (such as laxative tea during your cleanses) after using it for fourteen days straight, take a week break before continued use.

5. Salt Flush

(Refer to Challenge #6 for details on salt flush)

6. Oxygen colon cleansing pills

These are NOT the same as herbal colon cleansers. Sometimes they come in handy to bypass trying to strengthen and activate a sluggish colon. Sometimes we need to temporarily drop some TNT in the hole and blow the blockage away. (Sounds dramatic, huh?) That's when we can use oxygen pills.

How they work: As the magnesium-based powder is dissolved by the water, tons of pure oxygen and ozone is released into your colon. That literally oxidizes the hard, caked-up fecal matter.

Have you ever seen a compressed oxygen flow used to burn a hole in plastic? (Envision how the heat of the flame melts away candle wax.) It's exactly like that. It simply turns solids into liquids and gasses. Softens stools. Similar to the way that water is a universal solvent to dissolve compounds, pure oxygen (not just air) is highly potent AND safe for the body since only inorganic matter is affected by it.

TIP: These pills are to be taken at night, and they work while you're sleeping. So don't take the pills then do something like a salt flush right afterwards. That's washing the pills out before they can do their job!

7. Jogging

Jogging? How does that work to flatten internal gut waste? Imagine you have a large sealed bowl of Jell-O in your hands (I have no idea where I come up with this stuff) and you start jogging with it. What happens to the Jell-O? It get jostled and bounced and agitated. Same stuff is going on with the old gunk in your belly. (You runners might be thinking about the big poops you have after a long run, now.)

TIP: Low impact running machines (elliptical, etc.) do NOT have the same effect. You never create jarring motion landing on your feet with low impact machines. Try jumping rope or hula hooping, too.

REMINDER: Envision in your mind's eye what's going on here. Flexible tube in your body. Clogged with some soft, some hardened fecal matter. "Loosen that spaghetti."

PART 5:

WHAT TO EAT AND HOW TO EAT IT

The Slight Edge

Don't freak out, but I'm about to give you the single most important secret to a successful life. No big deal right? Really! This single concept, philosophy, thought process, view of the world has helped me to consistently make the right decisions for my career, relationships, health, EVERYTHING, since I was fortunate enough to be exposed to it.

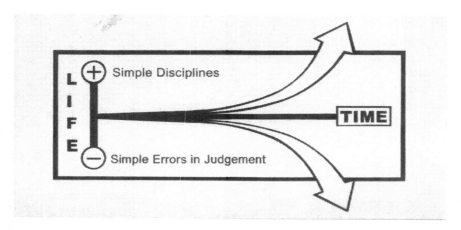

I read an amazing book by Jeff Olson called *The Slight Edge*. It helped me realize it's not those few BIG decisions in life that make or break us, it's the small ones that we make each and every day, hundreds of times a day. Those are the ones that compound over time to eventually take us on a path to seemingly magical success – or on a blameful path of failure.

Do I eat the bagel for breakfast TODAY? Do I take a walk after work TODAY? Do I take the stairs or the elevator NOW? Do I order the side salad THIS meal? Do I buy the gallon jug of ice cream NOW? Do I pick a date to start my Reset Challenge NOW? Over and over, we make these little decisions all day long. THESE are the decisions that compound day after day, week after week, month after month, year after year.

A PENNY A DAY, DOUBLED FOR A MONTH. If you were offered $1,000,000 (one million dollars) right now, or a penny a day, doubled *each day, for one month, which would you choose? One penny doubled every day for a month adds up to $10,737,418 and 24 cents. Compound interest. Leverage. Doubling. Geometric growth. It all adds up and that's YOUR SLIGHT EDGE.*

- **Success** (career, family, health, life) is achieved by simple daily disciplines repeated over and over.
- **Failure** is achieved by simple errors in judgment repeated over and over.

The trick is that slight edge decisions are easy to do (hit the gym instead of watch TV, order a salad instead of fries, drink an extra glass of water). But they are also easy NOT to do. How many times in the past week have you decided AGAINST one of those three things?

Another trap to not fall into is trying to see results right away. The guy that eats the McDonald's Big Mac is not going to immediately have a heart attack and die right? (That would certainly curb those 10 billion sold signs). He doesn't. And the person that ate a salad before their meal isn't going to have their grey hairs turn dark right on the spot or have their precancerous cells just pop out of them onto the ground, will they? NO.

Most of the time it's not about making the scary lifelong commitment to being healthy, it's about making a healthy decision right in that moment – a slight edge decision.

6 Rules to Eat By

I don't know about you, but I find it amazingly mind boggling how complicated it is to "eat healthy." Every month it seems that some new food is now good. Or it's now bad. Cooking this way is bad now. Combining this food with that is better than combining this food with that food. THIS color of some vegetable is way better than THIS color of the same vegetable.

And then how about all the darn nutrients on the labels? Sodium levels. Sugar ratios. Calories per serving (how big is a serving anyway?). Saturated fats vs. monounsaturated fats vs. polyunsaturated fats??? Chicken vs. beef vs. pork, etc.

Then what time of day to eat? How many meals per day? Drink water when you eat or not? Is it grain fed or cage free? Should you stand up when you eat? Sit down?!?!?

Ugh!!!!! This is just darn ridiculous, right?

At what point in human history did you need to a) have a legitimate degree in nutrition or b) be told by experts how to eat…food?

It doesn't seem to make sense right? I mean how do you think previous generations made it without the Internet and Dr. Oz? Those poor people must have been just overwhelmed by the countless options right?

NOPE.

Short answer:

Human beings eat two things 1) plants and 2) animals. That's it. If it's not a plant or an animal, your body has not evolved over the past 200,000 years to properly digest and assimilate it. Chemicals, preservatives, coloring, artificial flavor, etc. Those. Things. Are. Not. Food.

Only plants or animals. GOT IT?

(These examples are not all inclusive. Just a start – and my personal favorites)

Breakfast food examples:

- Eggs (whole egg. Not just egg whites)
- Bacon, sausage (no additives)
- Oatmeal (not flavored/ not pre-mixed packets)
- Fruits (not cans or cups)
- Yogurt (healthy bacteria!)
- Herbal teasBlack coffee

Breakfast NO-NO's:

- NO breads (toast, bagels, muffins)
- NO baked goods (waffles, pancakes)
- NO cereals
- NO milk (unless it's raw AND you want to GAIN WEIGHT)
- NO flavored coffee

Lunch & Dinner food examples:

- Meat (chicken, steak, fish)
- Vegetable salad (raw)
- Vegetables (steamed, sautéed, etc.)
- Brown rice (not every day)
- Wraps (tortilla)
- Vinegar-based salad dressings

Lunch & Dinner NO-NO's:

- NO breads (buns, sandwiches, biscuits, etc.)
- NO pastas
- NO creamy salad dressings (Ranch, Caesar, Thousand Island)
- NO french fries (the potato part is fine – it is the deep fried oil part that is bad)
- NO pastries (cakes, pies, cookies, etc.)
- NO processed frozen meals (typically with more than ten ingredients and added chemicals; ESPECIALLY diet meals)

Snack food examples:

- Fruits (apples, grapes, bananas, avocados, etc.)
- Vegetables (carrots, cucumber, broccoli, etc.)
- Nuts and seeds
- Whole snack bars (contains the full entire nut/fruit)

Snack NO-NO's:

- NO candies
- NO processed snack bars

Drink examples:

- Water
- Coconut water
- Herbal Teas
- Non-dairy milks (almond, rice, etc.)
- Fruit and vegetable juices (no sweeteners or chemicals added)

Drink NO-NO's:

- NO soda
- NO energy drinks
- NO flavored coffees
- NO milk (unless it's raw and you intend to gain weight)
- NO powdered drink mixes (Kool-Aid, Crystal Light, protein powders, whey, etc.)

So many rules, right? Great-grandma didn't have all these rules, right? Darn right, she didn't! Great-grandma didn't just jump in a car and to the drive-thru to eat every night. She had to make it herself. You know how long it takes to fry chicken? Bake a cake from scratch? And most of the above drinks didn't even exist! DID. NOT. EXIST.

***Obviously, on your cheat meal (once or twice a week) EAT WHATEVER YOU LIKE!! Break the rules. It's okay.

That's the short answer to how to eat. Now get out of here and start one change at a time! Don't try to revamp your diet overnight.

Keep a food journal of what you eat every day. Take a picture of each meal BEFORE you eat it.

Now here's the long answer (only for those that want to know WHY?):

Rule #1 – Eat only plants and animals, as close to their natural state as you can (not processed)

Why? That's what your human body has evolved to consume.

Apple vs. canned applesauce. [Apple wins]
Eggs vs. Egg Beaters. [Eggs win]
Pork chop vs. hot dog. [Pork chop wins]

Are there bad fruits or vegetables? NOT IN MY OPINION

Rule #2 – Avoid processed carbohydrates

Why? They swell up in your digestive tract and slow down digestion and they cause bulging in your intestines resulting in a protruding belly. They are also very far from the grain that they started as (what plant does it look like to you? Right.)

- NO breads (white, wheat, muffins, buns, French toast, pancakes, etc.)
- NO pastas
- NO pastries (cakes, cookies, pies, etc.)

Rule #3 – Avoid boxed and canned foods

Why? To prolong the shelf life of these products, they are stuffed with chemical preservatives and lots of the natural fiber is removed from the food (as well as anything that will rot). Not so natural anymore.

Rule #4 – Avoid overcooked foods

Why? Raw (uncooked) is always better if possible. The more we heat and cook plants and animals, the more live enzymes we kill off.

Steamed broccoli (four minutes) vs. baked broccoli casserole (steamed wins)

Raw almonds vs. smoked almonds (raw wins)

Rule #5 – Shop at health food stores and farmers markets ONLY!

Why? It lowers your chances of buying bad food. Put some trust in the store you're in. They aren't perfect but it's better than your standard grocery store.

Rule #6 – One or two cheat meals every week. (ANY ANY anything you want!)

Why? Because otherwise you'll quit! Plus 1 or 2 meals out of 21 meals in a week is nothing in the grand scheme of things. EAT UP!

Are you going to die if you break any of these rules? NO! But it's not going to help you get any healthier either.

Believe it or not, this food confusion has not been a dilemma on the planet Earth forever. As a matter of fact, this has only been an issue for the last 50 or 60 years or so. Yep, only the past two to three generations of us have had so many new food options. REALLY! We simply didn't have the technology or the motivation to use human ingenuity to create these amazing food processing options that allow us to make food last longer, stay "fresher," be so portable and convenient.

What changed?

Well there was this little skirmish called World War II in the 40s. Necessity was the mother of invention. We found a way to feed those few million troops overseas and the resultant food technology exploded from there. Make more food from less. Make it last longer. Make it cheaper. Check, check, and check!

So the solution to eating healthy mostly lies somewhere in the generations BEFORE WWII, right? But what? They ate meat and burgers and butter and pasta and candy just like us. What's the deal? There must be something subtle going on.

What else is in today's food?

Human beings eat two things: plants and animals. That's it. If it's not a plant or an animal your body has not evolved over the past 200,000 years to properly digest and assimilate it. News flash time: read the ingredient label on a box or can of something in your kitchen, a box of cereal for instance. I guarantee you that there are more than just plants and animals on that label, my friend. The ingredient in question was derived from a plant/animal originally (see the label to the left) but through physical or chemical processes, so much has been removed from the original source for reasons of texture or shelf life or coloring, etc. The final proportions of nutrients are no longer recognized by your body as a plant or animal. If I took at $100 bill and ran it through a shredder and tried to use those shreds to buy something, I'd have a rude awakening at the checkout counter. That's the same exact scenario going on in your body when eating processed foods. Worry less about the "Nutritional Facts" label and more about the "Ingredients" label.

Now What?

It's going to be inconvenient to eat a real, natural, healthy diet. America's current food landscape leans more towards convenience and storage than natural and healthy Accept it and get used to it. Stop waiting for some magical force to do it all for you.

You'll probably need to drive a little further to the health food store. You'll need to circle around the block a few times to find a restaurant that gives you the options you need. You'll need to trash a lot of the items already in your fridge and replace them with better alternatives. ("I'll finish what I already have so that I don't waste it." BULL CRAP you will. That stuff is fake food. Waste the hell out of it. It's wasting you from the inside out every time you eat it. Clean out your kitchen.)

Your friends will make fun of you and tell you that you are crazy and that you are wasting your time.

TIP: Be careful who you accept advice from. If you take their advice, you take their lifestyle.

Stick to your guns. BELIEVE that you are making the right decision and watch your body start to improve as you do. A few minutes of inconvenience will gain you years of energy and happiness beyond your dreams.

Don't forget to cheat!
This isn't an exercise of deprivation!!

Water

Have you noticed that I talk about water a lot? My buddy, Mark, jokes with me that my universal solutions to all problems are a) drink more water or b) read a book. I'm a simple man.

I've covered everything about why water is the #1 single most important change most people can make to their lifestyle in the Water Challenge section of this book. So taking all of that into consideration, I'm going to get all scientific on you.

People talk about "drinking fluids" as opposed to drinking water, including juices and sodas and broths, and milk, etc. What magical thing is water able to do that none of these other fluids seem to be able to do?

Water simply doesn't behave like other liquids. PERIOD.

- It is the only natural substance found in all three physical states at the temperatures that naturally occur on Earth. (Gas, liquid, solid = water vapor, water, ice)
- If you drop an ice cube into a glass of water, it floats. This happens because water expands as it freezes, which makes the solid form less dense than the liquid. But most other liquids do just the opposite; they shrink and become denser as they freeze, so the solid form sinks. If water behaved that way, ice in lakes would freeze from the bottom up (no ice skating)!
- Another surprising characteristic of water is that it boils at a very high temperature – 100 degrees Celsius at sea level – compared with similarly sized molecules. If water behaved like other liquids, it would exist as a gas at the temperatures and pressures found on Earth, and life as we know it couldn't survive.

- Another unique property of water is its ability to dissolve a large variety of chemical substances. It dissolves salts and other ionic compounds, as well as polar covalent compounds such as alcohols and organic acids.

Imagine all those weird, beautiful, unique things water does inside your body in your miles of veins and in your organs! We see water so much and are so surrounded by it we really take it for granted. Now go get a glass of water!

I prefer to have it at room temperature (as opposed to with ice cubes) so my body doesn't need to waste energy cooling it down or heating it up. Plus it's easier to chug room-temperature water. Feel free to squeeze some lemon juice in your water for more flavor and to help fight acidity in your body. NOTE: those little lemon shaped bottles of "lemon juice" at the grocery store are NOT fresh lemon juice.

Can you drink too much water?

It hurts my heart every time I run across an online article or some medical "expert" that is hell- bent on scaring people by yelling at them that they are harming their body by drinking so much water. As well intentioned as these individuals may be, they are missing one crucial thing: common sense. We've evolved on this planet for millions of years. We are NOT surrounded by a poisonous substance (water) that is toxic to you. They say it depletes our cells of sodium. This is partially true which is why I use sea salt liberally on my food to replenish any lost minerals. They claim that it overtaxes the kidneys. Water? Don't you mean chemical-laden juices and energy drinks and sodas and alcohol? If you've lived a few decades with bad eating habits, making your organs (kidneys included) weaker and less effective, the Reset Challenges are designed to flood those organs with oxygen and water and remove all the waste so they can operate as they are designed to.

With the increased toxic load of the times we live in, we need to constantly go a little bit above and beyond to remove toxins that we haven't evolved to deal with (jet fuel, smog, fluorine, chloride, food preservatives, etc.).

It's like trying to start an old lawn mower that you haven't used in years. It's been sitting out in the rain and in the elements, rusting (yep, that's your innards). The first couple of cranks on the starter cord won't do so well, will they? Add some more gas. Try again. Add some oil. Try again. Spin those blades by hand. Try again. Voila. The LAST thing you want to do is give up and leave the mower for dead.

If you drink too much, you'll pee/sweat it out, along with any toxins encountered. DON'T. GIVE. UP. And be patient as the process works itself out.

What type of water is best?

So now we agree that water is good, right? But there are 9 million types of water. The question always pops up, which one is best? Trust me, I get it, and I was confused as heck years ago too. Spring water vs. filtered water vs. distilled water and so on and so on. Remember these two things:

1. Companies profit by selling a product that they can differentiate from other products
2. Any water is better than no water.

This list is my rating, in order of most preferred to least preferred. But remember, any water is better than no water.

Filtered Water – This water has been passed through a fine strainer or charcoal. It removes solids and preferably chlorine and fluoride from the water. (Those chemicals were added to the water so it could travel from the water treatment plant in your city, through miles of pipes, to your faucet without being infected by every bacteria and germ along the way. Live in a major city and you want tap water without some sort of filtration? Drink Mexican tap water then get back to me).

Spring Water – This water is from an underground source. Assuming it's authentic, this is pretty chemical free and still has a natural amount of minerals in it.

Distilled Water – This water has been turned into steam so that all of its impurities are left behind and then condensed back to liquid. This water has no minerals in it and tends to be slightly acidic. This is best for cleansing, as it leeches minerals and toxins from the body (great for the short term, not great for the long term, in my opinion)

Reverse Osmosis Water – Similar to distilled water in that this water is stripped of all of its minerals.

Alkaline Water – Also called ionized water. This water is made by using very strong magnets to effectively split water in two. You drink the highly alkaline water (acids have lower pH, bases have higher pH. 7 is the middle – neutral pH) and it's supposed to keep your body from becoming acidic on the inside, thus preventing sickness and disease. My only issue with that is that instead of digestion and assimilation causing cells to be alkaline, we are just pouring highly alkaline fluid in the body and that might neutralize stomach acid.

Bottled Water – This water can be any type of the above waters.

Tap Water – This water tends to have chlorine and fluoride in it. You're not going to get sick after drinking a glass of it, but keep in mind that those chemicals add up glass after glass, day after day, year after year. A great experiment is to shower with tap water and note how dry and tight your skin is. Then use a quality shower filter and notice how you don't need any moisturizer after that shower. That's happening on your insides too!

Garden hose and park drinking fountain water. As a child that grew up drinking out of these, I can attest to the fact that you're not going to die or get dysentery if you need to have a drink on a hot day.

"I want to fill my belly" is the wrong way to think.

--Fills belly--

Rice

Bread

Pasta

Also clogs digestion and expands the belly.

"I need high energy, live food" is the right way to think.

--High energy--

Uncooked vegetables

Uncooked fruits

Try a high-energy diet for two weeks and see how you feel!

Check out the rules for the 21 Salad Challenge!

You will read many articles online that will scare the crap out of you about viruses and bacteria in these different types of water. I don't doubt their validity. I'm just not afraid enough of germs to freak out. Make your own choice.

Sea Salt

Man! This is honestly one of my favorite topics. I'll give you a hint. Nine times out of ten, if the media and mainstream medicine are against some sort of food or treatment, I will probably love it and do my BEST to go against the grain. Why? 'CAUSE THE MAINSTREAM AIN'T WORKING! Too much obesity and cancer and heart disease and diabetes. (Many of you will fight me on this and cite how your doctor has been warning you for years to cut salt and sodium from your diet. Relax for now. Try to understand this other perspective first. Then make your decision after seeing for YOURSELF.)

So let's talk about salt and sea salt. We got hosed! That's right. Years ago, someone made a conclusion that sodium is a health issue and started the trend of no salt and no sodium and we have been suffering as a nation ever since (same thing happened with the guy that said eating fat was a killer). Frick and Frack, these two clowns!)

Fact: These are the four most important elements needed for life:

1. Oxygen
2. Water (not technically an element – but you get the point!)
3. Sodium
4. Potassium

So you remember that we are made up of trillions of cells, right? And you remember that water is pretty important stuff. What if you have great oxygen intake and you're drinking tons of water. That should be all that you need to hit the critical needs, right? Actually, not completely (I know, I know. It never ends, does it?)

If you tried the Water Challenge, you may have noticed that you peed A LOT with the addition of all that water. You most likely need to add some more sodium (in the right proportions – sea salt) to complete the formula. Then voilà! Your cells are actually taking advantage of all the precious water now. (Now don't go thinking that you wasted your water during the Water Challenge if you peed a lot and didn't have any sea salt. Believe you me, you benefited your body TREMENDOUSLY.)

We need to make sure that the water actually makes it through the cell membrane and INSIDE the cells. That's where sodium becomes so very important. Sodium is the gatekeeper of water for cells.

There are basically two seas of water in your body: 1) the sea of water OUTSIDE of your cells and 2) the sea of water INSIDE your cells. The OUTSIDE sea is supposed to have a higher concentration of sodium than the INSIDE sea (that proportion controls how much new water gets through the cell membrane and into the cell).

So just throw some more table salt on there right? Oh, if it were only that easy! We humans had to go and muck up salt too!

What would a caveman do? He'd consume salt in its natural form by exposure to seawater.

The highest amount of sodium in nature is found in seawater (92 minerals).

Incidentally, this is the SAME exact proportion and balance of minerals as found in the body.

Table salt has two minerals, sodium and chloride (NaCl). They removed and bleached out those other 90 minerals, which means table salt has WAY too much sodium, proportionally. Remember that the puzzle pieces need to combine in the right order and the right proportions to complete the puzzle and THEN your body can recognize what your putting in your mouth as food and do the right thing with it. Well, in this case, our "puzzle" has too many corner pieces (sodium and chloride) and nowhere near enough middle pieces.

What salt is good salt?

Himalayan Pink Salt and Celtic Salt have about 80 minerals in them. You can find them at any health store and very easily online. Natural salts like these will NOT be pure white. They will look brownish or pink or something other than just stark white. How natural would stark white salt from the earth be?

How much?

Use sea salt liberally on your foods and when you're cooking. I DO! Stop being afraid of it; be natural with it. And you don't need to freak out if your only option at that meal is table salt. With your high level of daily water intake, you won't do yourself any harm with that table salt. I would MUCH rather you use table salt instead of using NO salt at all (as long as your water intake is high). That sodium is important.

What happens when people get enough water and enough sea salt?

Check out www.WaterCure2.org. It has countless testimonials of people that increased their water consumption and sea salt intake and cured their asthma, alcoholism, arthritis, cancer, diabetes, high cholesterol, chronic fatigue, colitis, Crohn's disease, depression, anxiety, diabetes, fibromyalgia, and obesity.

Do I think sea salt is the magic panacea? No. But I do know that cells need OXYGEN, WATER, AND WASTE REMOVAL to thrive and live indefinitely. Sea salt helps to complete that formula and the cells take it and run from there.

Don't be 1 of the 19...

Fruits and Vegetables

So your goal is for 70% of the food you eat to be plant based. Why not just go vegetarian? Well, at the time of writing this book (see how I'm open to possible change!), I believe that we as human beings have evolved on a planet that has very available meat options. I can't imagine a scenario where our caveman relatives would pass up eating a tasty deer or a wild boar (assuming they caught one that day). But I can see them mostly eating plants since they are a lot less mobile and they don't fight back.

With that said, I have noticed major performance increases in athletes when sticking to a vegetarian diet ON GAME DAY. They eat their normal servings of meat the days before and the days after, but upon rising on game day, they avoid meats and dairy until after the game. Why?

1. Digesting meat takes a lot of energy. Your body is basically deconstructing the food to get all the way back to the energy that it came from: the sun. Sun →Plant →Animal →Human
2. Your weak spot will suffer while this high-energy process is happening. Got bad joints? You'll feel it more when you

eat meat. Got asthma? You'll feel it more when you eat meat.

I recommend you try it out on your own. See what your results are and make your own balance of plants and animals.

Every month I receive a different newsletter touting the latest super vegetable that is the "one veggie you need to make you healthy and burn all your fat and prevent cancer." Sadly, my dear friends, Super Plant is about as real as Superman. Yes, it's absolutely true that different vegetables have different healing effects on your body. For sure:

- Tomatoes are great to help lower blood pressure.
- Pumpkin seeds are great at reducing inflammation in the prostate.
- Parsley is fantastic at helping with bladder infections
- Carrots help correct poor eyesight.
- Kale is killer for detoxing cells.

On and on and on. But here's the trick. You can't just eat one and be done. The trick is to eat them all. Think of it this way: all those plants are able to heal some malady, right? So instead of using them to heal something you have, why not use them to prevent that disease. If from the time you're born you are constantly eating a wide range of vegetables and fruits – ones that lower blood pressure, others that improve eyesight, still others that help poor eyesight, etc. – you can effectively PREVENT those ailments just by constantly ingesting the cure. The ultimate vaccine, huh?

I believe that the vast majority of plants on the planet are able to provide some sort of medicinal benefit to the animals on earth. Plants are here to heal.

Cooking Vegetables

In the 1930s, Paul Kouchakoff, M.D. showed that if you ate a diet that was more than 51% cooked food, your body reacted to the food as if it was being invaded by a foreign organism. Think about that: cooking alters food so much your body thinks it needs to defend itself! Here's the save. He further demonstrated that if 51% of your meals were raw you would have no leukocytosis (no white blood cell reaction), so your immune system would not be activated with a false alarm. Ah ha!

So what rules can we take from this for cooking vegetables?

1. Less is more. No need to pre-cook/sauté vegetables then add them to our recipes
2. Steaming is better. Get a vegetable steam tray. Steam veggies for no more than four to five minutes
3. Never boil vegetables. You're basically making vegetable soup. Then you pour away all the nutrients in the water!
4. Eating salads with your meals helps your body have fewer immune system reactions

Keep in mind, these are simply targets. Will you end up cooking vegetables for longer? YES. Will you die because of it? NO. Just keep these rules in mind and you'll be fine.

Animals – Meat

In the past decade, these poor creatures have been blamed for the entire downfall of human beings and our health!

- "Countries with high consumption of animal-based foods in 1983-84 were more likely to have higher death rates from 'Western diseases.'" – The China Study
- Red meat is bad for you
- More and more Americans are becoming vegetarians or pescetarians or even going vegan

"So what's the deal? Do I need to stop eating meat to get healthy and Reset my body?" NO. Not in my opinion. Remember me? I'm a traditionalist. I think that we have all of the evidence on how we need to live by modeling what has worked and not worked for the past 200,000 years of humans. Did the previous 7,000 generations of humans eat meat? YUP. Did they eat MOSTLY meat? NOPE

If all their lives they ate and lived the wrong way, they didn't have drugs and doctors so:

- If the food made them too weak, they would not have survived long enough to reproduce and raise offspring (bad habits died with them)
- If they were injured too easily – same thing
- If they developed chronic diseases – same thing

Important: We are the survivors. The best of the best of the human race. We are the product of the right lifestyle habits that helped our ancestors live while others died. Stop messing it up!

I personally eat meat 2-3 times a day. Here are my meat rules:

1. Eat organic, free-range meat WHEN POSSIBLE. That means if you have a choice, choose organic. That does NOT mean be "that guy" and turn your nose up if you are offered conventional meats. You can control what you buy when you grocery shop, but don't be rude to your family and friends. Remember: one steak will not kill you.

2. The less processed, the better. The less altered from its natural state the better. For example, grinding up tens of different cows and combining them to make ground beef is not as natural as a piece of steak. Blending and grinding pork, beef, and chicken trimmings, adding chemical additives and flavoring, and then wrapping them in a cellulose tubing to make a hot dog is not as natural as eating a pork chop.

3. Think about what went it to getting that meat to your plate. Turkey is not inherently better than chicken, which is not better than red meat. Where did that belief come from? They are all just animals, right? BUT "the man" started confining cows (to save space) and injecting them with antibiotics (to fight the resulting sickness) and feeding them growth hormones (to have more to sell) and feeding them corn instead of grass. Thus a less healthy animal and far less nutritious animal to eat. But then what

happened? Then they got to chickens – they never had a chance. So the thing that makes the meat more or less healthy is how healthily the animal itself is raised. Your food is what it eats too.

Fat, fat, fat!

One of the biggest screwups in American food history was the low fat thing. HOLY CRAP!

Your body sooooo needs fat. But now with everyone drinking low-fat and skim milk, low-fat yogurt, etc., we are getting nowhere near the healthy amount of fat that we need to run these bodies of ours. Think about it, milk doesn't come out of the cow that way, does it? There is a process to take the fat out of natural, nutritious, rich milk. How would a cave man do that?

Does eating fat make you fat?

HUH?! No. Does eating muscle give you muscle? Does eating hair cure baldness? HUH! You get the point. I eat as much fat each and every day as I possibly can. I eat at least one avocado every morning. I add a tablespoon of grass fed butter to my coffee. I snacks on almonds all day long, I cook with olive oil. I ALWAYS eat the fat on my meat. EAT YOUR FAT!

What started this low fat mania?

Back in 1980, a study was published concluding that eating lots of meat lead to high cholesterol and heart issues. But fearing retaliation from the meat industry, the USDA modified things to say that eating lots of FAT was the cause. Two years later the new guidelines were published and here we are today.

Why eat more fat?

- Better reproductive health. Guys – more testosterone. Ladies – more balanced hormones and estrogen production. Stronger libido – or as Marvin Gaye would say, "Let's get it on…."

- Better skin. The upper layer of skin is fat. No more dry skin. Smoother, softer, more uniform skin. You will need a lot less makeup and you'll look years younger.
- Better source of energy. As you Reset, your body will switch from burning sugar for energy to burning fat for energy (got any extra fat laying around?).
- Brain health. Your brain is more than half fat.
- Stronger bones.
- Better liver health.

How do you tell a "good" fat from a "bad" fat?

GOOD FATS	BAD FATS
Avocado	Margarine and other vegetable oil spreads
Butter (especially grass fed)	Processed vegetable oils Canola, Sunflower etc.
Nuts	
Coconut Oil	
Olive Oil	
Animal Fats	

Don't be 1 of the 19…

Soda and Energy Drinks

Remember the old television shows *Lassie*, *Leave to Beaver*, and *The Little Rascals*? (I just went waaaaay back on you, huh?) These shows were filmed back in the 1950s. They were about a bunch of American kids. Do you remember what they drank most of the time? Soda? Red Bull? Nope. Water. (And milk. A lot of milk. I'll cover that soon enough). Sodas were like the ultimate reward if the kids on those shows did something well. (Trust me, when someone threw those kids a nickel they bounced for joy to the nearest dime store.)

See the section in this book about the Water Challenge to see why water is the ONLY liquid that works like water.

Are you like me? I used to think that clear sodas (7-Up, Sprite, etc.) were healthier than colored sodas or colas. NO. It's the chemicals in the soda and the lack of water that is the issue. You can't see those based on the color of the dye used to attract you to it.

Do you have to give up soda and energy drinks to be healthy and Reset your body? NOPE. Not at all. Your body is not that weak that you can't treat yourself to a soda or a Red Bull a couple of times a week, but let's keep it at that. With your dramatic increase in water to offset the dehydrating effects of things like sodas and energy drinks, you will continue to help your body to remove any toxins every hour of the day that you are drinking water.

--How to eat--

Pick a meat. Pick a vegetable. Done.

You do not need a "starch." You do not need bread.

(Make sure it's not filled with chemicals)

Fast Food

Oh, you convenient scourge of mankind. Of all the things that we ALL know not to eat, fast food tops the list. It's amazing if you think about it. Fast food isn't even a single TYPE of food. It's just a way that food is prepared and served. ANYTHING can end up in the fast food category.

So let me be very clear here. NOT ALL FAST FOOD IS BAD. Most of it is. But NOT ALL FAST FOOD IS BAD. I personally eat at Chipotle fanatically (three times, at minimum, weekly). Most of their food is free range, natural, and clean. I LOVE IT.

So what makes fast food so bad? Honestly, it's only two things:

1. Too many chemicals
2. Too many buns

Organic Food

The funniest thing about organic is that probably 75% of the population doesn't REALLY know what organic really means.

A cow is a cow is a cow, right?

Not really. If you raise cow A on a farm and let it graze on grass and don't inject it with any drugs, and then you slaughter said ill-fated animal and grind the meat and put it in a supermarket is that the same as cow B, who was raised in a crowded pen and was not allowed to move and exercise? No sunlight. Living in its own poop. Eating corn (cows have not evolved to eat corn). The cow begins to get sick and diseased due to the poor conditions. So we inject the cow with antibiotics to keep it "healthier." We also want bigger cows so we inject it with growth hormones and steroids. Now the cow is juiced up and filled with yeast (yeast is the byproduct of months of antibiotics). Then we take it and grind the meat and mix it in with countless other cows and stick it in a supermarket.

Same?

Need I go on? And by the way, this isn't just about beef or meat or animals. You can also apply this to fruits and vegetables.

As I mentioned before, avoiding pesticide residue on foods is NOT my number one reason for eating organic food. The main reason I eat organic is because NON-organic food – animals injected with growth drugs and given excessive antibiotics and fed unhealthy foods – are less healthy themselves. Plants grown with chemical fertilizers and sprayed with pesticides and prematurely ripened using gases are less mature, less nutritious, less flavorful, less vibrant, less energetic, and less healthy. It's common sense. Our food is what IT eats too.

How does that affect the end result? Less flavor. Fewer nutrients. Fewer medicinal properties.

Think about this. For the vast majority of human history, agriculture could be described as "organic." Only during the 20th century was a large supply of new synthetic chemicals introduced to the food supply. The organic farming movement arose in the 1940s in response to the industrialization of agriculture and was known as the Green Revolution.

Ummmm. So food has been organic for the past few thousand years, up until about 70 years ago? Interesting....

"But the studies say there is no nutritional benefit to organic food!" Therein lies the problem. Our nutrient-measuring method does not accurately help us gauge how healthy food is AT ALL. Remember when I said food is not its sum nutrients? Science does not know how to take all the known nutrients in a carrot, pull a Humpty Dumpty, and put them all back together to CREATE a carrot. Right? It's those things that we can't measure yet – that we don't even know exist – that's the stuff that makes a food healthy. The energy in the food.

What if a race of super huge aliens tried to determine the nutritional content of human beings. (Yup – Terry went there!) These 1000-foot giants are comparing a super healthy person that has Reset his body for years to a highly overweight Standard American Diet person.

- Alien 1: "This small one has one heart, one liver, red blood, and a grey brain. What about the larger human?"
- Alien 2: "All the same here. This one has even more blood and a larger heart. Maybe it's healthier?"

No. I am not getting loopy. But really! Those basic observations DO NOT properly tell us if those two people are similarly healthy. Right? Who has more energy? Who needs less fuel to get the same job done?

Milk

Mooooooo. It does a body good, right? Kind of. Milk is a mammary secretion intended to feed and nourish young mammals before they are able to digest food on their own. It makes things grow.

- So if you can't digest food yet, drink milk.
- So if you want to grow and gain weight, drink milk.

If you don't want those things, then DO NOT drink milk. Milk isn't killing you, but it's not helping you lose fat either. So let's say you do want grow and gain weight (I drink two or three glasses of milk each day, with the intention of gaining weight). This is what you need to know:

Drink milk as close to its natural state as possible – stick your mouth under that udder and squeeze!

That means drink whole raw milk – milk that is not homogenized or pasteurized.

Homogenizing – When milk is whole, the cream naturally settles to the top. Homogenization is the process by which the cream and the milk are forcibly combined so they don't separate. So instead of larger milk molecules, you have much smaller milk molecules that a) make it harder to digest (lactose intolerance, anyone?) or b) is thought to cause scarring in arteries which leads to heart disease.

Pasteurizing – Heating milk up to 145 degrees for 30 minutes. Does it kill harmful bacteria and dangerous germs? YES. Does it also kill beneficial bacteria too? YES. Does it destroy some iodine in the milk? YES. Does it kill some of the very enzymes needed to help digest the milk? YES.

As I'm writing this, the sixth Google result for "pasteurizing milk" is an article from the FDA's website "The Dangers of Raw Milk." You mean the milk that comes, unprocessed, straight out of the cow? That stuff that humans have been drinking for thousands of years? That's dangerous (and even illegal in some states)? Come on!

The Tale of Two Calves is a thought-provoking experiment reported by Michael Schmidt that you can find on the Internet. They took two calves and five months later compared them after one was raised on raw milk while the other was raised on pasteurized milk. Amazing differences. The pictures alone tell an amazing tale of malnutrition. (This wasn't a full blow scientific study with thousands of calves. It was just two calves, FYI)

- The pasteurized milk calf wasn't growing fast enough (42% less than raw milk calf)
- The pasteurized milk calf had super smelly, runny, pale manure

After slaughter, the organs were almost night and day! (Pale kidney and liver. Stomach content was a MESS in the pasteurized milk cow)

The pasteurized milk calf's testicles were shriveled up and significantly smaller (pay attention boys!)

Is that little experiment saying that drinking pasteurized milk will make that happen in you? NO.

The experiment is implying (in this order):

1. The young need fully nutritious food to properly grow and develop.
2. Heating up natural food removes enough of its nutritional content to have a dramatically diminished effect on those feeding on it.
3. Pasteurized milk is not nearly as nutritionally powerful as raw milk.

Raw Snacks

Let's face it; you're going to get hungry between meals. I feel like I'm constantly sticking food in my face all day long. (I'm always trying to add more muscle and I stay very active – FEED ME!) So let's be smart and keep bad foods out of convenient reach and good foods as easy to come by as possible. Use our laziness to our advantage!

Good snacks to keep in the kitchen, at the office, and in the car:

Fresh fruit, fresh vegetables, dried fruit, almonds (and other nuts), sunflower seeds (and other seeds), baby carrots, bell peppers, cucumber slices, trail mix, kale chips, hummus dip.

Yet again, YOU MUST READ THE LABELS! Raw (uncooked) is always better than roasted/cooked versions. Keep an eye out for additives and "natural flavorings" (aka chemical shit storm). Visit the bulk section at the health food store and snack on those items. In general, boxed snacks are less fresh.

What about snack bars?

Less is more! Fewer ingredients. Less processing. Less, less, less!

Most have too much added sugar, canola oil, flour, "natural flavors," and a host of other processed, man-made ingredients.

The ultimate goal is to have a bar where you can see and identify the nuts, fruits, and seeds all in whole pieces – and it's all held together by some natural sticky/gummy material.

Probiotics and Cultured Foods

I'll be honest; I'm no bacterial biologist so I won't have all the answers and atomic-level knowledge to explain every single detail behind why probiotics and cultured foods are so critical for human digestion and health. But I'll give you a boat-ton of logic and common sense.

The classic definition for probiotics follows along these lines:

Probiotics are the beneficial microorganisms (bacteria and beneficial yeasts) that the body needs to promote healthy digestion, nutrient assimilation, and many other vital processes. The main job of these beneficial microorganisms is to preserve the natural balance of microflora in the intestines necessary for the proper digestion and assimilation of food.

What happens if you DON'T have a proper amount of that good bacteria in your gut? Crappy digestion, diarrhea, fewer nutrients extracted from the foods you eat, constipation, hard stools, bellyaches, bloating, flatulence, gas, etc.

TOP 8 PROBIOTIC FOODS to add to your daily diet

1. **Yogurt** – a starter culture of Lactobacillus bulgaricus is added to milk. That bacteria then breaks down the lactose, which benefits those lactose intolerant folks. It's worlds apart from drinking milk. It's far better to eat yogurt even if you just want to avoid weight gain from drinking milk. Just be sure to read the label to ensure the yogurt has "live cultures" or "live organisms." Lately, Greek yogurt has gained the reputation as the "good yogurt." Don't get caught up in the hype. Read the label to see if it's good or not.

2. **Sauerkraut** - Made from fermented cabbage. Any type of cultured vegetables will be great. Easy to find at a health store.

3. **Kefir** - Similar to yogurt, this fermented dairy product is a unique combination of goat's milk and fermented kefir grains.

4. **Miso Soup** - Miso is one the mainstays of traditional Japanese medicine and is commonly used in macrobiotic cooking as a digestive regulator. Made from fermented rye, beans, rice, or barley. Adding a tablespoon of miso to some hot water makes an excellent, quick, probiotic-rich soup.

5. **Kombucha tea**- This is a form of fermented tea that contains a high amount of healthy gut bacteria. I love

them. Try to find one that still has the "mother" at the bottom of the bottle (it's a web like substance).

6. **Pickles** - Believe it or not, the common green pickle is an excellent food source of probiotics. The less commercialized the better, but most pickles will have some microbial value.

7. **Kimchi** - An Asian form of pickled sauerkraut, kimchi is an extremely spicy and sour fermented cabbage typically served alongside meals in Korea.

8. **Probiotic Supplements** - Chewables, powder, capsule, liquids. Holy probiotics, Batman! There is much debate as to which of these forms is actually THE BEST. Chewables: Too processed – skip 'em. Powder: Some say they don't make it past the stomach's harsh acids to get in the lower intestines where they need to work. Capsules: Some have delayed- release capsules to resist stomach acids. Liquids: Many say these are the best and the freshest of the probiotics, especially if they are kept refrigerated. My verdict? EXPERIMENT! I've tried them all and I go back and forth (right now, I'm on the liquid supplement party train).

You have this final wave of soldiers in the lower part of your gut, and their job is to complete the digestion and assimilation of the food that has made it all the way through your stomach and small intestines, to pull some vital nutrients and prepare the waste to be excreted cleanly and painlessly. Help your gut, help YOU!

And if you're female (hey, ladies!), then you have a bonus reason to keep your healthy bacteria count nice and high...your vagina! There are millions of live microorganisms in your vagina and when the bad guys start to outnumber the good guys, Candida yeast can cause pain and discomfort.

Ever taken a dose of antibiotics for an infection? The good news is, those antibiotics probably did a great job of killing off the harmful bacterial infection. The bad news is antibiotics are more like a bazooka than a sniper as a weapon. They will kill any type of bacteria, including some of your beneficial, good bacteria. That's why doctors recommend women eat yogurt when taking antibiotics. So be sure to increase your probiotic food intakes during and after any antibiotic doses.

Cooking

COOK MORE! It's that simple. At least once a day. Try to cook at least 10 meals per week. If you eat three times a day, that's 21 meals per week. You will have FAR more control of the food and the ingredients that end up in your body.

Don't know how to cook? Get a cookbook. Experiment. You eat three times a day. There is NO EXCUSE for not knowing how to cook my friend. Take a cooking class. Burn a few things. Just practice, and you'll get better.

Travel too much? You always have a choice. Find a way to travel less. Your job might be killing you. You don't HAVE to work that way. Just decide what's more important for YOU in the long run.

Too busy? Slow the hell down! What's more important than your health? What's more important than having more energy and vitality each and every day to help you get things done? What's more important than being the best you can be?

You don't like to cook for just yourself? Cook for your neighbors and friends. Cook multiple meals for the week. GET OVER IT! Create an imaginary friend and have a date night!

They say that human beings are the only living things that prevent themselves from reaching their full potential. Have you ever seen a tree that didn't grow as tall as it could?

Microwaves

In early 1991, word leaked out about a lawsuit in Oklahoma. A woman named Norma Levitt had successful hip surgery, only to be killed by a simple blood transfusion when a nurse "warmed the blood for the transfusion in a microwave oven"!

Have you heard of the experiment where the student has plant A and plant B. She microwaves water to a boil, then cools it and waters plant A. And she stove heats water to a boil and cools it and waters plant B. Over the next week, plant A dies!

Why are you NOT supposed to microwave baby's milk? It's been known since 1989 that it converts many of the amino acids and fatty acids to substances that are poisonous to the nervous system and kidneys.

Why did the Soviet Union ban the use of microwave ovens in 1976?

Microwave ovens use electromagnetic energy to basically excite the molecules deep inside the food, especially water molecules, thus creating heat. MAGIC! So what's the problem? Well, over the years, incidents like the ones above got people thinking. Have you noticed that microwaved food – even coffee – will taste less flavorful and rubbery versus food heated on the stove? Why is that? Heat is heat is heat, right? Think about it. They don't just taste different for no reason.

In 1991, a food scientist who had been fired from a major food company published a research paper that described how *microwaved food became "denatured." It changed the molecular structure enough to make your body react to it as if it were a foreign invader.* Blood samples of the volunteers in the study degenerated within minutes of eating the microwaved foods even though conventionally cooked foods had no such effect. Interesting. Are we letting convenience and new technologies slowly rob us of the very gains in health and life expectancy each generation?

I threw my microwave oven out seven years ago. "Oh my heavens! How do I heat up food now?" USE. A. STOVE! Use a covered pan with some water or oil in it on the stovetop. Use a covered pan in the oven. I PROMISE you that taste improvement alone will keep you doing it. Unplug your microwave, put it in storage, and make a decision to improve your health!

Reading Food Labels

I distinctly remember, years ago, laughing hysterically at the thought of reading my food! I'm pretty sure I said aloud, "I will NEVER read my food. I'm not that desperate, bored, or anal. Give me a break!" Ahh, how those words taste in my mouth today!

The sad truth is that in this day and age, you HAVE to read the food labels. Why? Because it's not the food that's really the problem, it's the stuff IN the food that's the problem. Every company is trying to make their product stand out from the next guy so that we gullible consumers buy it. That's how they make money. They are not necessarily trying to be evil and destroy the health of their customer base (I don't like conspiracies), BUT they are being socially and morally irresponsible by playing to people's "right to choose." AND no one just ups and dies when they eat the food, so it's honestly hard to directly connect the poor health to the meal they just had.

Food Label Rules

1. Pay less attention to the nutrition facts label and more attention to the ingredients label.

- Nutrition fact labels list out calories and nutrient breakdown per serving size (sodium, fat, vitamin A). In my opinion, that's pretty useless information because those numbers are including any effects of the chemicals, drugs, or additives added to the food too. I can't digest and assimilate that stuff. Why do I care about its nutrients?
- Think of it this way. Gold. If I'm trying to see how valuable a clump of gold is, I measure it, right? I have two boxes each with a clump of gold in them, box A and box B. Box

B weighs more so that box is more valuable, right? What if I open box B and not only is there a clump of gold but there is also a bunch of sand in there? Is box B still more valuable than box A? No way. Sand just added to the weight, not the value of the box. Nutrition fact labels basically just measure the "weight" of all the junk in that box of food (the food you can actually digest and every other bit of "sand" added to it as well). The ingredients label tells me what's in my box. What is really "gold" and what is really useless "sand" that my body will need to fight through to make use of that "gold."

2. Order of ingredients

- The actual ingredients are listed by order of weight. So the first thing listed is the most abundant in that food. If sugar is listed first, RUN!

3. Number of ingredients

- Generally, less is more. Some say five ingredients or less. That's a bit overgeneralized, but you get the point.

4. Bad things

- In most cases, if you can't pronounce something on the label, you don't want it in your body. Sugar, high-fructose corn syrup, MSG (monosodium glutamate), PARTIALLY HYDROGENATED OIL, POTASSIUM BROMATE, FOOD COLORINGS. Bad, bad, bad.

This is by no means an all-inclusive list (think dictionary-sized book for that) but it's a start.

Medicinal Foods

I believe that our Earth's ecosystem has spent billions and billions of years to maintain an equilibrium. It's self-sustaining already. That means for everything that happens, there is some equal yet opposite thing that counterbalances it. We won't run out of anything and we won't have too much of anything in the long run (of course, we overly intelligent humans have been messing with that balance for the past two thousand years or so. Trust me, the planet will figure out a way to get back on balance and it ain't gonna look pretty for a bunch of us!) But I digress…
On a small scale, it's like this:

- Bird kills mouse
- Mouse remains are on the ground
- Ants swarm and consume carcass
- Microorganisms finish the job, reducing remains to dust
- Dust settles into dirt adding nutrients
- Plant grows and feeds on that new fertile dirt
- So on and so forth for years….

Another part of that balance is that most every plant provides some sort of medicinal benefit to animals. It's the ying and yang.
I try to include foods with the strongest antiviral and antibacterial and anti-inflammatory properties into my daily diet. Why? An ounce of prevention is worth a pound of cure, right? No need to heal from a cold if you never get sick.

Here is a list of my favorite medicinal foods:

Garlic – I eat one clove of this every morning and one every evening. It's one of the most powerful antimicrobial foods you can eat. Eat more if you are sick and want to heal exponentially faster! Add to soups and salads and marinades and meat spicing.(Great for viral infections, cold sores, herpes, HPV, flu, etc.)

Ginger – I make tea out of this root a few times a week and sweeten it with honey. Works in minutes to settle stomachaches caused by bad food. You can just bite off a thumbnail sized piece and chew for a few minutes to get the juice and swallow a glass of water to get it in your stomach. (Ever wonder why it comes on the side when you order sushi? Wink wink.)

Onion – Order onions on everything! Such an easy way to stay germ-free. On salads, wraps, burgers, in eggs, soups, etc.(also great for viral infections).

Turmeric – This root also does a great job at fighting and preventing inflammation (aka swelling. Any disease ending with "-itis" means it is caused by some sort of inflammation (arthritis, bronchitis, etc.). Sprinkle turmeric powder on your veggies, add it to your soups, eat curry chicken. You can also buy it as a supplement.

Lemons – Did you know ancient Egyptians believed lemons were effective against poisons? They are highly alkalizing once processed by your body (even though they taste so acidic). Squeeze the juice into your water, add to your salads, and make lemonade from scratch. (NOTE: Don't use the processed, fake lemon juice in the plastic lemon bottle)

Coconut Oil – Use this for your cooking oil, add this to your coffee, and eat a spoonful every day.

Fermented Foods – Pickles and olives and pickled veggies, etc. I snack on these daily. Keeps the beneficial bacteria in your gut nice and high. (Digestive issues BE GONE!)

Prunes – My personal favorite belly-flattener food. Super-high levels of fiber keep you regular and in and out of the john in record time!

Pineapple – Now you have a reason to visit a tropical island! Great part of a breakfast fruit salad.

Honey – Honey contains an enzyme that releases hydrogen peroxide, which effectively kills off certain kinds of bacteria. Use in your teas.

Cabbage – Makes for a great salad or cabbage soup.

18 - 24-Hour Cycle

FACT: 300 billion cells die and are replaced every day in the human body. 300,000,000,000…with a "b"! What does that mean? Well, what are those 300 billion new cells every day made of? Whatever you ate that day, my friend (wink wink). Those are the building blocks for construction. Did you eat a large bag of Doritos? Hopefully, it wasn't heart cell day. Did you chow down on a pint of ice cream? Of course it wasn't brain cell day, right? Don't freak out and don't be scared. It's not permanent – every three to ten years all of your cells are replaced anyway. And every day you have the opportunity to choose what you build yourself out of that day. You always have a choice.

When you go to sleep every night (or take naps), your body does most of its repairing and rebuilding. Every night when you are sleeping, all the energy you aren't using to move and think and see is all being diverted to heal damage and create new cells. That is where the magic happens.

A healthy person should pee very light, yellow pee if they aren't dehydrated (strong yellow or dark pee = Drink More Water!)

A healthy person should have 2-3 bowel movements per day, 20 minutes after each meal. (Where do you think all the food goes??)

A day in my mouth

I wake up around 7 a.m. I brush my teeth with a mixture of 40% baking soda & 60% sea salt on my toothbrush. I rinse it out with two capfuls of hydrogen peroxide. Then I chug a tall glass of filtered, room-temperature water. (I cut and squeeze half of a lemon into it.)

Then I pour a glass of whole, raw milk. I lay out a few scoops of yogurt to snack on while I prepare breakfast: three pasture-raised, organic eggs, seasoned and scrambled with chopped onions, mushrooms, cheese. Two slices of bacon on the side along with a whole avocado with sea salt sprinkled on. I chomp down on three or four prunes. (I eat a lot, huh?)

I grab a medium, dark roast, black coffee on the way to the office (sometimes I plop a couple of teaspoons of grass-fed butter in it for more fat and creamy flavor). I bring a bag with me to my office (a banana, a grapefruit, and an apple). I snack on them until lunchtime.

Lunchtime: I head to a Greek/Mediterranean restaurant for steak or lamb skewers and a salad. Or a restaurant that has sandwiches that they will make into a wrap for me. I add a side salad to it (constantly ordering "off menu"). Sometimes I'll have a coconut water afterwards.

During the day, I'm snacking on pickles, almonds, and dried cranberries. I chug a couple of tall glasses of water.

At the end of the day, on my way home, I stop at the health food store (unless I'm lucky and it's farmers market day) and grab fresh food for the night. At home, I'll make a delicious stir-fry with seasoned chicken or pork and bell peppers, snow peas, bean sprouts, mushrooms, onions, and garlic. Or I'll grill up a mouth-wateringly seasoned steak and steam a huge pan of broccoli liberally sprinkled with sea salt.

I have another couple of prunes, a couple of slices of pineapple. I'll chill out and read for a bit and have a glass of red wine.

Sound fancy and totally unrealistic based on your current eating routine? I KNOW! This would have been **my version when I was 30 years old:**

Wake up at 8:30 a.m. Pop 4 Eggo waffles in the toaster. Drink some overly processed orange juice or eat a bowl of cereal. Or stop at Jack in the Box for a breakfast sandwich with hash brown wafer. Then lunch was any hamburger and fry combo meal. (I rotated between the fast food places daily.) Have a sweetened ice tea or fruit-flavored sugar drink. Snack on potato chips and/or a Little Debbie snack cake during the afternoon along with a Red Bull drink. Dinner was a box of Hamburger Helper with a can of green beans. And washed it all down with sweet tea or Kool-Aid.

Why do I tell you this? Because this Reset isn't theory. I had to break over 30 years of bad habits to make this work too. It took seven years to get where I am now (it's not overnight) but I tracked and noticed improvements and results EVERYDAY so I was encouraged to stay the plan.

If I can do it. You can do it. You deserve it.

PART 6:

WHAT TO DO WITH YOUR BODY

"Anyone who lives a sedentary life and does not exercise, even if he eats good foods and takes care of himself according to proper medical principles — all his days will be painful ones and his strength shall wane."

Maimonides, treatise of Hygiene 1199 A.D.

Hot damn!! You're eating right, you're drinking right. We have 80 percent of the equation dialed in now. Ready for the secret sauce that accelerates all of the magical results? These are the things that will help to Reset your body that don't involve food and drink. These practices are like adding nitroglycerine to your race car's fuel to accelerate your results. Burn the fat faster; build the muscle faster; purge the toxins faster; heal your body's weak spots faster!

Exercise

Yup, I waited until the last section of the book to talk about exercise. Does that mean that exercise is not important? NO. Exercise is critical. You will NOT effectively remove toxins and slim down or improve your body's health completely without exercise. Period. You will be able to make great gains. You will be able to burn off tons of fat and tons of toxins without proper exercise, BUT you won't be able to do it as quickly or as thoroughly or as aggressively as many will need (after years and years of neglect). I've seen many people totally change their health and shed hundreds of pounds and beat cancer and change their body's shape JUST by changing their eating and drinking habits and cleansing. For sure!

What about the flip side? What if you did a ton of exercise BUT you never worked on the fuel that you're putting in your body? What if you hit it hard at the gym and CrossFit and your sport but you never removed the years of already-present toxins in your body that are keeping you running at 70 percent of your energy and health potential? Then you would be running an uphill battle EVERY DAY. You'd be using WAY too much energy to get the same thing down. You'd be fighting your body's organs with your muscles. That's a battle your muscles won't win.

What is the purpose of working out?

Stimulate your body's muscles to expand and contract. Activate your body's lymph system to remove cellular waste. Create slightly jarring movement to dislodge impacted intestinal material. Force your cells to scavenge fat reserves. Force blood flow into unused body parts. Improve body flexibility and blood flow. Prevent atrophy (use it or lose it).

Core Reset Step #8 is to work out 4 days per week.

Questions:

What is considered a workout?

Physical activity that makes you move your body constantly for 30 minutes. (You may need to start slowly). Hiking (level street walking is not a workout), jogging, a sport, Wii Fit, climbing stairs, weight lifting, cardio activities, hula hooping, jumping rope, calisthenics (jumping jacks, sit ups, etc.), heavy yard work, boxing, karate, aggressive dancing, boot camp workouts, P90X (and other workout videos), swimming. There are plenty of others.

What is NOT considered a workout?

If you have doubt that something is a workout, it's probably NOT a workout! (e.g., golf is a sport, but it's not a workout in and of itself. You don't think Tiger Woods got all his muscles by swinging a club and walking eighteen times in three hours, did you?!) Push yourself. You're only cheating yourself.

What if I already have been working out?

Even better! CHANGE your workout immediately. Your body is totally used to whatever you've been throwing at it — bored even. Like to do weight training? Get a trainer and have them mix it up! Like to hike? Do some different trails! Like doing home workouts with videos? Get a whole new set of DVDs and change it up.

What if I have an injury?

This will be true for lots of you (and me) since our bodies were in a weakened state for years. Start slowly and do things that don't cause pain.

Got a bad back? Try stationary biking, hiking (walking helps to alleviate back pain), swimming, elliptical type machines. There are many others. Get creative!

Got bad knees? Try those hand peddling bikes, upper body weight training, calisthenics, kettle bell swings.

NOTE: I don't like knee braces because they artificially hold your knee in place. It's important to use and gradually strengthen the tiny muscles in the knee. Same with wearing orthotics in your shoes. It temporarily relieves the pain but it weakens the joint even more over time. Have you ever had to wear a cast for a broken bone for months? How weak was that body part when you finally took that cast off? Same thing happens with knee braces and orthotics.

JUST DON'T GIVE UP! Your body is trying to heal itself. Be patient and track your improvements no matter how minor they may seem. It means it's working! The day will come when your injury will NOT stop you from the workout/sport that you love. BELIEVE IT!

Walking

How boring is walking?! I know, I know. But crazy as it sounds, human beings are totally designed to walk. If you think about it, a normal person (normal fitness and no injuries) can pretty much walk forever. Give them some comfortable shoes (or barefoot if walking on grass), find a way to feed them on the go, and what's stopping them other than sleep?

SO DO IT!

Lymphatic System

One of the most important benefits of walking is it activates your body's lymph system, the garbage collection unit of your cells. Your body has two major circulation systems: blood system and lymph system.

Blood – Carries nutrients and oxygen to your body's cells. It is pumped around by your heart.

Lymph – Removes and carries waste and toxins from cells to your lymph nodes to be eliminated from the body. (There is two to three times more lymph fluid in the body than blood.) It only allows lymph fluid to move in one direction away from the cells and it has NO PUMP. As you move, gravity drives the circulation of lymph fluid.

You need to take a 20-minute or longer walk EVERY SINGLE DAY! You can't miss a day on this one, gang. Letting those cellular toxins build up all day, then falling asleep and giving them another eight hours to do who the hell knows what inside your body ain't a good idea! Sometimes taking a walk outside might be especially inconvenient (blizzards or unsafe weather, temporary intense work schedule, etc.). Many will keep a rebounder in their home or office in those cases. It's a mini trampoline (it was the first thing I bought when I started Resetting).

Takes about 15 minutes to walk a mile.

Got an errand to run that's a mile away or less? WALK!

That's walking distance.

(Bonus – you'll kinda feel like a tourist in your own town!)

Too cold? (Bundle up!)

Too hot? (Bring some water!)

In a hurry? (Do it during the walk!)

Legs hurt? (Walk around the block!)

Stop making excuses and get your arse out there!

How do you use a rebounder?

- You don't need to work up a sweat to benefit from rebounding.
- Come up on your toes then drop back down. That's the light bounce that you need to benefit from rebounding
- You don't need to jump in the air while rebounding. Just bounce from toe raises.
- 15-20 minutes is a great rebound session
- It's important to be well hydrated (makes more lymph fluid)

Men: To help decrease your risk of testicular cancer, it's recommended that you wear loose fitting boxer shorts while rebounding to allow unrestricted movement. (Things that don't move don't circulate lymph well.)

Women: To decrease your risk of breast cancer, it's recommended that you rebound without a bra, if possible.

Breathing

WAIT! Don't skip this section. Yes, you know how to breathe. (I'd argue that you're doing it right this second!) What I want to talk about now are some techniques that you can use to increase the primary element used by your 100 trillion cells to stay alive longer. Oxygen.

We've already established that oxygen, water, and waste removal are the basic needs to keep cells alive indefinitely, right? See how long you can hold your breath for again. So how do we get more of the pure, precious, energy-giving oxygen deeper into our bodies, deep where our most starved cells need it most? Heart cells with more oxygen make a better heart; brain cells with more oxygen make a better brain.

Let's put this all in perspective: Every time your heart pumps, it's pushing around between 1 to 2 gallons of blood and it does this 60 to 80 times per minute. The more oxygen you can have in that blood, the more oxygen can make it to your cells. Think about what happens to the parts of your body furthest from your heart if a) there is not enough oxygen left in your blood by the time it makes it there (cold, numb fingers and toes are a possible sign) or b) if your heart is too weak to push hard enough to get blood to those faraway areas as frequently as needed.

Do you think that you're taking in 1 to 2 gallons of air when you breathe in?

FACT – Most people only use about a third of their 2.5-liter lung capacity

How to breathe properly:

Most of us spend our entire adult lives breathing incorrectly. We take in short, shallow breaths that don't fill up our lungs and don't fully oxygenate our blood.

- Breathe in through your nose – Your nose hairs and mucus are designed to catch and filter any contaminants in the air. Use 'em!

- Breathe from your diaphragm, not your chest – Best way to practice how this feels is to lie on your back, put your hand on your belly, and focus on breathing deeply so that your belly rises.
- Take as deep of a breath as you can, every time – Yogis believe the life span of a person is measured by their number of breaths. If a person's inhalation is rapid (think how a rabbit breathes), he will die younger. If a person is economical with their breath (think how an elephant breathes), they will live a hundred years or more.
- 5 seconds – Breathe in slowing and smoothly until your lungs fill to capacity
- 5 seconds – Exhale slowly and completely
- Do that for five minutes, twice a day.

Heads up, you might start to feel a little light-headedness the first couple of days when you practice this. It will pass. Stick to the plan.

Barefoot

Ever heard of Earthing? I'll give you three guesses what planet it was invented on. It's a super fancy way to describe walking barefoot and grounding your body to the Earth. "Why does anyone care about that? Why, why, why?" Remember, I'm always in the pursuit of what a caveman would do? I'm convinced that everything that our bodies have adapted to over the past 200,000 years affected us in a certain way and is partly responsible for us still being here today. NOTHING IS RANDOM and the devil is in the details.

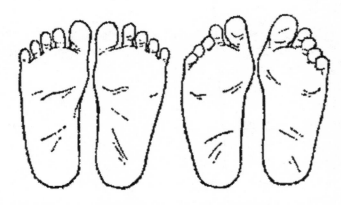

NATURAL FEET AND TOES BEFORE
WEARING MODERN SHOES

FEET AND TOES AFTER
WEARING MODERN SHOES

Which feet do you have?

Why I go barefoot as much as possible:

- We weren't born with shoes on! (Use that logic on wearing clothing as well.)
- We walk differently with shoes on. Pay attention to your body. It's very subtle, but your foot strikes the ground differently.
- Why? Simply put, shoe soles are not as flexible as the bottom of a foot, so instead of each part of your foot

reaching the ground milliseconds after the other in an unconsciously controlled symphony of orchestrated muscular/tendon/bone movements, your foot is strapped down to a flat surface that changes the timing of when the front and the back of your foot reach the ground (To exaggerate the effect, think about walking around wearing skis. Can you say awkward?)

To me, "walking differently" is the same as "walking incorrectly."

- Shoes weaken feet – Have you ever had to wear a cast? Do you remember how weak your arm or leg was after the cast was removed? Your muscles shrank. That's the same type of thing that happens to your feet after keeping them supported and immobilized in shoes. Use it or lose it, they say. What's even worse, in my opinion? Wear orthotics or wedges in your shoes. They totally weaken the muscles in your feet. They might hold your foot in place temporarily and give you some pain relief, but as soon as that shoe comes off, reality returns. The answer is to strengthen the muscle, not baby it.

- Shoes deform feet – Fallen arches, compressed toes, and bunions can result from how a foot changes shape after being confined in shoes for as little as one to two months as a child.

- Shoes change how your ankles and knees and hips work – Your leg, from the bottom of your foot to your waist, has three different pivoting, angling joints (ankle, knee, hip) that are constantly bending and flexing to compensate for the moving world around them, including all the joints below them. Think about it – when the angle of your foot changes, your knee then needs to adjust a bit. When your knee bends differently, your hip needs to adjust a bit.

- Those minor changes in angles compound over the years to lead to joint issues higher up the leg.

- You need to discharge built up electricity in your body. How often do you actually touch the planet Earth? Not your shoes touching ground. Not your feet touching carpet or concrete. How often do your feet touch dirt or sand or grass? That's the Earth. Have you ever built up an electric charge by sliding your feet across a carpeted floor and then touched a metal door handle? ELECTRIC SHOCK!

Think of that process going on and on for days, weeks, months until you actually ground yourself with the largest magnet we have, the Earth.

Ideas:

- Never wear shoes at home
- Walk barefoot on grass or sand every week for 20 minutes
- Wear flip-flops instead of shoes, when you can
- Wear minimalist shoes (e.g., Vibram 5 Fingers)
- Walk on your toes to strengthen your arches a few times daily
- With your feet flat on the ground and aligned straight (outer edge of feet parallel), squeeze your entire foot (as if trying to grip a branch as a monkey would). Hold that for three seconds. Relax and repeat ten times a few times per day.
- As you walk, consciously keep your feet from pointing outwards or from pigeon-toeing inwards. Keep the outside edges of your feet parallel to one another. Correct the angles in your foot muscles and ankles and knees while walking.
- You may notice temporary cramping and slight pain in your feet and joints. That makes sense, right? We are forcing some changes in the lifelong functioning of your joints. It will take some time to get used to it. But it's worth it in the long run. I'm flatfooted. And because I don't have an arch, I basically walk on the inside of my arch, which pushes my big toes in, which thus crowd my other toes outwards. That also makes for bunions, which is just a fancy term for the joint of the big toe over protruding

(eventually it can cause a lot of pain when walking). I'm 40 years old. Do you think that if I do nothing, by the time I'm 60 that bunion will be better or worse? What about 80 years old? Worse is right!

I take action NOW so that years from now, I'm not suffering. It's worth it!

Sweating

Why is "Sweat for 15 minutes weekly" a core Reset Step? Because you can sweat out as much toxic material in one hour as you can pee out (with a healthy set of kidneys) in an entire day. ...YUP!

Benefits of sweating:

- Clears skin
- Removes internal toxins

Ideas to work up a sweat:

Sauna

- My #1 way to sweat every week. Infrared or conventional dry sauna.
- 140degrees – 160 degrees
- Stay in the sauna for 10-15 minutes at time
- Stay hydrated (you need to be hydrated so you can sweat the toxins out. Drink up!)
- You can take a super cold shower in between steam room/sauna sessions to maximize your detox. (Heat brings blood and toxins to the surface. Cold sends blood deep into your body and organs. Always end on cold.)

Steam room

- Stay in the steam room for 10-15 minutes at time
- Stay hydrated (you need to be hydrated so you can sweat the toxins out. Drink up!)

- You can take a super cold shower in between steam room/sauna sessions to maximize your detox. (Heat brings blood and toxins to the surface. Cold send blood deep into your body and organs. Always end on cold.)

Yoga

- Heated yoga or Bikram yoga will be the best to get an awesome detoxification. As you are performing the poses and stretches, your internal organs are literally being wrung out (like a wet towel) and toxic material is seeping out of them into your bloodstream and out via your sweat/ (Stay hydrated so that you don't just free up a bunch of toxins and feel sick!)

Outdoor work

- In the olden days, it was called working. Yard work, chores, gardening, jogging, etc. On a nice hot day, get out in the sun and work up a sweat!

Sex!

TIPS:

Your pores will be wide open after your intensive sweating. Be careful what you put on your skin then because it will be absorbed quickly. Avoid chemical-laden soaps and lotions. Afterwards, simply rinse off, dry off, and be off.

Hot and Cold (Hydrotherapy)

Let's make some blood magic happen! This a super powerful way that many have used for thousands of years to cure disease, remove internal waste, feel invigorated, and deliver an energy burst to your body.

Why it works:

Your blood has critical nutrients needed by EVERY part of your body. Unfortunately, a weak heart, blockages, poor circulation, tight clothing, and injuries can prevent those critical nutrients from reaching some parts of our body or not enough is getting there to make a difference. This is the fix! The importance of the alternate use of cold and heat lies in the fact that heat stimulates the surface areas of our body and increases blood supply to the skin, while cold stimulates blood circulation in our internal organs. Alternating heat and cold makes the circulation move in and out like an accordion. This has the effect of unblocking stuck flows.

This is how to do it:

1. Make sure that the water used does not contain chlorine, fluoride, or other highly toxic chemicals commonly used in public water supplies. It is counterproductive to greatly increase one's circulation and at the same time drive in a large dose of toxic chemicals. If you cannot readily filter these chemicals out of the water before it comes into your home, install a showerhead filter that is truly effective in this regard. Home Depot sells some that use replaceable carbon cartridges for about $30.
2. Get completely wet with a temperature of water that is comfortable.
3. Slowly increase the temperature to the point you can barely stand it. Quickly expose all the parts of your body to this hot water, including the top of your head and your face, for 40 seconds.

4. Now turn the water temperature down to the coldest tolerable setting. No matter how cold the water is at its coldest, it cannot harm you in any way. The only thing stopping you from going to the coldest setting is your ability to confront the experience. Make sure all parts of your body are exposed for 20 seconds.

5. Next, turn the water to hot again but make it a little hotter than you had it before. Again, get each part of your body good and hot before reversing the temperature to the coldest setting for 40 seconds.

6. Repeat the procedure seven times – seven times hot, seven times cold. Always begin with hot and end with cold. Make the temperatures as hot and as cold as you can tolerate. Be sure not to scald yourself.

You will notice an amazingly pleasant tingling all over your body that can be described as "feeling squeaky clean on the inside"…so, so good!

Regular Water Immersion

There are people out there that haven't taken a bath in years! I don't mean they haven't bathed, they shower daily, BUT they have not immersed their body in water, literally, in years. There are apartments and houses that don't even have bathtubs anymore, just showers. "Well, I still get clean, Terry. What's the big deal?" I'll tell ya what the big deal is. Five words. What would a caveman do?

Each organism begins its life in water; a human fetus is no exception. Kneip, a German physician, wrote, *"Each contact with water means an additional minute in our life."* How do you imagine that our pre high-rise tower dwelling ancestors cleaned themselves? What about the fact that, before the use of oil to make transportation exponentially easier and faster (the past 100 years or so), humans lived EXCLUSIVELY near bodies of water in order to survive. The first oil well was in 1859 – 155 years out of 200,000.

To put that in perspective: one tenth of one percent of a full year = 6 hours. Think about all the events you went through in the past year. Can you capture all of your habits, highs, lows, benefits, shortcomings, of that year by looking at a six-hour block for a single day?

What if you happened to be on vacation during the six hours we sampled? That's not a good reflection of how your entire year turned out. With that same thinking, what have we, as humans been doing with the other 99.99% of our existence?

So, put your entire body under water regularly.

Benefits of water immersion:

-   Allows more water exchange into your skin (better skin and body hydration)
-   Expedites scar/injury healing
-   Helps to cleanse and promote vaginal health
-   Promotes removal of toxins through the skin
-   Clears pores
-   Keeps skin tighter
-   Reduces wrinkles

GET WET!

How?

-   Bathe at least once a week (the more, the better!)
-   Swim (In the ocean is the best. The natural salts detoxify and cleanse your body like no other!)
-   Hot bath with sea salts (excellent for detoxifying)
-   Epsom salt bath (helps reduce muscle soreness – removes lactic acid build up)
-   Hot tub (the fewer chemicals, the better. Try ozone and other alternatives as a sanitizer)

Skin absorbs EVERYTHING!

Amazingly enough, the vast majority of us are living in denial. I know I was for years. "My skin doesn't absorb things on it. That's crazy!" Yet, if I was foolish enough to write on myself with marker or a pen, I could see it start to fade (as my skin ate it up). How do those nicotine patches work? What about birth control patches? Why do we rub ointment on insect bites? Because it gets into our bloodstream (regardless of what you've heard). Common sense, right?

Try this little trick: Rub fresh garlic on your feet. You'll taste it in your mouth within the hour!

Women absorb up to five pounds of damaging chemicals a year thanks to beauty products.

Will wearing some moisturizer kill you today? NO

Will applying some base and some lipstick kill you today? NO

Just keep in mind many contain man-made chemicals. Those are toxins. Does your body like toxins?

Benzoyl peroxide is found in many beauty and skin care products. It does a great job of temporarily improving skin appearance, for sure! And a little bit of the toxin is absorbed by your skin. Then you put it on the next day…and the next…for a week…a month…a year. It builds up.

A rule of thumb: If you wouldn't eat it, don't put it on your skin.

If I placed a liter container of benzoyl peroxide in front of you, would you drink it? Well, that much will build up with days and weeks and months and years of use. Believe it.

No need to freak out and be afraid of everything in your bathroom cabinet. BUT, be aware and start to replace those NONESSENTIAL products with more natural, less processed alternatives. After replacing each product as the opportunity arises, you'll gradually assemble a very clean, very healthy collection of products that you are soaking into that lovely skin of yours.

Frequently used products to be mindful of:

- Lotions and moisturizers
- Hand soaps
- Body soaps
- Facial soaps
- Hair shampoo
- Hair conditioner
- Makeup
- Lipstick
- Hair perm kits

Don't laugh, but I used S-Curl (a hair relaxer) until I was in my 30s. After thinking more about the chemical shit storm going on in my scalp every three weeks, I let that lifelong habit go (and I still think I'm pretty cute without it!)

Don't be afraid of the sun

"Get out in the sun, and get some vitamin D!" How many times have you heard that one? You'd think that Mother Nature is doling out multivitamin pills. Of course being in sunlight helps your body to produce vitamin D, thus preventing lots of nutritional deficiencies. But is that it? Will taking a vitamin D pill replace your need to take a walk on a sunny day? Here's what I think.

All on life on this planet starts with the sun somehow:
Sunlight → Plants → Animals
No sun, no plants, no animals. (You're an animal, silly!)

Do you notice how more motivated and energized you feel on a sunny day vs. a cloudy day? Even if it's not warm outside – you skiers and snowboarders know what I'm talking about.

It's ENERGY. Energy that we can't even see is firing off the sun at the speed of light. Million and millions of joules of energy.

We set up solar panels to clumsily convert that precious light into useable electricity (plants have been using sunlight to feed the world for billions of years).

Being in the sun every day gives you energy.

What about sunburn and skin cancer? What about my pale-skinned brethren? One word: moderation.

As vital and life-giving as energy from the sun is, it's a VERY strong energy source. Too much of anything isn't good. For example, fire: a light stove flame to boil some water vs. a house-engulfing inferno!

Listen to your body and use the shade if you need to to keep from turning a good thing bad.

Sunscreen or not?

Americans are obsessed with sunblock. We are so afraid of the sun, we set timers to remind us to reapply sun block when outside. People are constantly poking one another and timing the fading of the pink discoloration. (Having a built in tan, I still don't know how long is too long for the pink to fade.)

What if we've made it for the past 200,000 years without needing sunblock? What if our poor diet and lifestyle and addiction to antibiotics (known to cause higher sunburning) are weakening our skin to the point that what used to be "normal" sun exposure is too much for our thin skins now?

What if applying more and more chemicals to our skin (which we know will be absorbed into our bloodstream) is causing more toxic overload and all of the side effects that come with it – skin damage, skin cancer, skin aging?

Sunscreen Alternatives:

- Eat more good fats (the top layer of your skin is a thin layer of fat)
- Eat more berries and grapes (studies show less UV damage in hairless rodents – YUCK)
- Apply sesame seed oil every one to two hours
- Apply coconut oil every hour
- Apply aloe vera every one to two hours

Herbal Supplements

Now we're going to talk about some ways to hack into your body's natural reactions and dial them up or dial them down WITHOUT any man-made chemicals, medications, or side effects. Sadly, I didn't invent this stuff. Older humans than I figured this stuff out, literally since the beginning of human history.

I believe that the vast majority of plants on the planet are able to provide us with some sort of medicinal benefit. Plants are here to heal.

"I've tried herbs and they didn't work!" "I need something that works faster!"

There are two reasons people have these complaints:

1. Their bodies' systems are not in sync yet. Too much clogging from a low-energy, highly processed diet. Herbs work by stimulating your body's natural systems. If your body is too out of whack, the effect of the herbs is far too little, far too late. They basically bounce off your body and get peed away. (Imagine your body is a city, and we're trying to drive a package across town. If there is no system to transport things around – roads, stoplights, snow removal, etc. – that car isn't going to get very far, very fast.)

2. The herbs are too weak. Either the dose isn't enough or the potency is too low (weak plants).

Imagine your body is that same city with good enough transport systems, but now, the car you're in doesn't have enough gas to make it across town!)

Step one is to make sure that you are Resetting your body and flushing out old waste and helping your systems to communicate better. Increase your cellular strength by following the **13 Core Reset Steps** so that your body's systems are working together as they are designed (get your body's transport system working). Then you need to make sure that you use quality herbs. Just like any other product in the world, some are better at their job than others (be sure your car has enough fuel to get the job done).

Step two is to do some research and find herbs that will help with your body's weak spots:

- Bad joints? Try – Turmeric, Fish Oil
- Low on energy? Try – Yerba Mate, Ginseng
- Got bad eyesight? Try – Bilberry, Eyebright
- Skin issues? Try – Aloe Vera, Witch Hazel
- Constipated? Try – Castor oil, Senna
- Headache issues? Try – Feverfew, Lavender, Skullcap
- Digestion issues? Try – Ginger, Mint
- Trying to fight a cold? Try - Echinacea, Garlic,
- Fighting a yeast infection? Try – Oregano, Grapefruit Seed Extract, Tea Tree
- Want to even out your insulin? Try – Cinnamon, Cumin
- Want to kick-start your liver? Try - Milk Thistle, Burdock root,
- Want to clean out your kidneys? Try – Dandelion, Alfalfa
- Herpes or cold sores? Try – Ginger, Garlic
- Bacterial Infections? Try – Echinacea, Garlic,
- Want to alleviate premenstrual tension? Try – Black Cohosh, Dong Quai, Wild Yam Root
- Prostate issues? Try – Saw Palmetto, Pygeum
- Want more sex drive? Try – Women: Damiana, Shatavari. Men: Yohimbe, Horny Goat Weed
- Want to fire up your brain? Try – Gingko biloba, Ginseng, Rosemary
- Soothe an insect bite? Try – Lavender, Calendula

There are literally THOUSANDS of different herbs that have natural enhancing effects on your body to give you the little leg up that you need to take full advantage of your body's supremely working systems. There even different ways to take those supplements:

Plant form – You may know them as spices. You've been cooking with them all your life. Pepper (improves blood flow), turmeric (reduces inflammation), parsley (diuretic to relieve bloating), etc..

Teas – You can grab them in bags already chopped up OR you can get the raw herbs, put them in a boil ball, and make a medicinal tea. Ginger tea with honey is delicious. (Teas are weaker medicinally than infusions and extracts.)

Powder/Capsules – This doesn't require any heat overprocessing. The herbs are basically chopped up and then packed into a dissolvable veggie cap. You can pull these pills apart and pour out the powder inside. No heat needed. No binders needed.

Essential Oils – These are made by steaming plants and condensing the vapor back down. They are SUPER concentrated (e.g., one drop of rose essential oil contains 60 whole roses!)

Tablets – These are the hard pills that you would need to chop to make smaller. They have to be heated (remove the moisture) and combined with binders ("pill glue") when created. That can introduce unwanted/unneeded compounds AND lower the potency of the herbs (heating).

Extracts/Tincture - The body does not need to break down a liquid extract, allowing more of the medicinal properties to be absorbed into the system. This makes an extract much more powerful than a capsule or tablet. These are the liquid versions of herbs. Liquid extracts take one to four minutes to assimilate.

In order for any nutrient to reach the cells of the body, it must first be suspended in a solution. Or in other words, it must be liquid. As a rule, the nearer an herbal preparation approaches the liquid form, the quicker and more completely it will assimilate and take effect in your body.

It is ALWAYS better to ingest a strong tea or a tincture. Tinctures (being alcohol based) absorb through the stomach into the bloodstream immediately and effectively. The only time this is NOT desirable is when the herb is being used to heal or treat the digestive tract.

"But my doctor says herbs don't work!" Does that even make any sense? We already know that different foods have different effects on your body's systems (lemons will prevent and cure scurvy, coffee beans make you pooh afterwards). Laboratories have the patent on affecting change in the body? I think not. Don't believe them. Don't believe me. Experiment and find out for yourself!

Naturopathic Doctor

Let's get started building you a team of experts! This isn't a one-man show, nor will you need to be a lone vigilante all your life if you have some ailments that you want to address. Consider the next few people I'm going to talk about the same way that the president considers his cabinet of advisors. The advisors are all experts in their areas, with years of experience under their belts. The president gathers their opinions but, at the end of the day, the president makes his own educated decision as to what course of action to take. He's the Man. You're the Man (or Woman)!

First, find a naturopathic doctor that you can trust. Some naturopathic doctors are completely anti-drug, some will use them in extreme cases and then get you back on track naturally once the beast has been beaten down enough. (Maybe you've had an intense disorder for years and they will medicate to get it under control and then put you on a more sustainable path going forward. That's EXACTLY what drugs and medication are for). Some will talk about oxygen therapy (cool stuff!), ultraviolet blood work, vitamin C injections, energy healing, and all sorts of other procedures you've probably never heard of. (Don't be one of the 19 anymore!)

You can use the Internet to find them, ask trusted friends, visit your local farmers market, health food store, hippie festivals. (Really!) Go where they will be. Get out of your old preconceived notions. Think differently. Be open to new ideas. Do what the other 19 won't do.

DO THIS EVERY DAY!

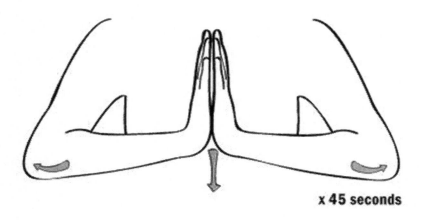

x 45 seconds

When I was a computer programmer in my 20's, I started noticing carpel tunnel symptoms. I started do this stretch every day for 45 seconds. It went away in one week. DO IT! (I use the steering wheel of my car to stretch against on my commute to work!) Why?

1) Typing shortens the muscle under your forearm, so stretch it to lengthen it back (it ain't magic)

2) I wanted to be preventative so that when I was 40 (as I am now), I wasn't hating life! START

"If you do a little bit now, you don't have to do a lot later"

Chiropractor

These poor guys get such a bad rap. "It's only a temporary fix!" "You get hooked and have to keep coming back or your problem returns." Every heard or said any of those?

How does it work?

In oversimplified terms, different parts of the spine control different organs and different areas of the body. Your spine sends electrical signals to them to control their regular functioning. Think of the spine as you would an old-school phone switchboard. Each time a message needs to be sent to a part of the body from the brain, this controls message distribution.

No arguments there, right? So the chiropractor's job is to keep those channels of electricity unobstructed and clear so a full, strong signal gets to where it needs to go. He does that by adjusting varying parts of your spine (oversimplified).

I remember my first adjustment. I had already been Resetting my body for a few years, so I had pretty open, well-working systems, so I gained maximum benefit from this alternative treatment. For two days after that first adjustment, I had some interesting reactions. Within the first hour, I had a huge bowel movement, and I felt as if I had a cold (Herxheimer reaction). Then a week later, I had another adjustment and another huge poop after that one. What was going on? Apparently, my body had been experiencing a blockage. After the adjustments, those channels opened up and set off a toxin chain reaction. It was a rather cool experience! I have a monthly adjustment, preventatively. I want my electricity flowing very freely to my organs, thank you very much!

Yes, it's temporary!

Why? Because you keep messing it up!

Every day that you sit folded up in a chair for eight hours a day, it causes damage and smashed up nerves.

Every night that you sleep in some unnatural position, it causes damage.

Every time you do some wild workout move that you haven't warmed up for, it causes damage.

You screw up your spinal signals all day long. What's wrong with taking five minutes to fix them every few weeks?

"It doesn't work on me!"

Most likely, your body systems are still not in sync yet. Too much clogging from a low-energy, highly processed diet. If your electrical energy is too low or your systems are still too backed up and not communicating well yet (keep Resetting), the adjustment is basically too low-impact to have an effect. (Imagine your body is a city, and we're trying to drive a package across town. If there are no systems to transport things around – roads, stoplights, snow removal, etc. – that car isn't going to get very far, very fast). Don't fret. Just keep Resetting. Give it time. NEVER GIVE UP!

How often?

Your chiropractor will know what's best for you. Based on my athletic lifestyle, my clean eating habits, and my weak spots, once a month works for me. It's literally five minutes of adjusting and about fifteen minutes of warm up on a warm back massager.

Starting off, you're probably going to need to go at least weekly and then gradually space out your adjustments to your long-term frequency (every 2-4 weeks).

Massage

They feel so good! Why don't we get them more often? I do! I get a 60 to 90 minute massage every 2 to 4 weeks. I love it!

Benefits:

Eases sore muscles, reduces pain, improves sleep, and boosts immunity

You're milking toxins out of your muscles and skin. You're helping blood flow all over your body. You're stimulating your lymph system to pump toxins out of your cells.

There are soooo many types of massages: trigger point, Swedish, deep tissue, sports, etc. Get any kind that you like or want. Just get them often and regularly. Fully-clothed massages? DO IT. Oils and lotions? YES and YES. Five-minute chair massage at the airport? GO FOR IT.

Go ahead, make an appointment now!

Does it hurt when you sit cross-legged?

You probably also have bad knees or lower back pain!

Tights hips – from sitting a lot – effects the joints above and below the hips:

your knees & your lower back.

LOOSER HIPS MEANS LESS KNEE & LOWER BACK PAIN. REALLY!

Try these hip stretches daily. (Hold each stretch for two full minutes!)

And sit cross-legged more.

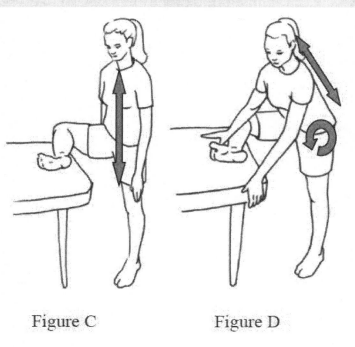

Figure C   Figure D

Reflexology

I'll admit it took me a while to come around to this one. But man, oh, man, do I use it often now!

Years ago, when I began Resetting and I was working on my poor knees, I had a man I affectionately refer to as the Witch Doctor work his magic (he was a chiropractor by trade, but he also incorporated deep tissue work, herbal healing, and muscle testing, and he consulted a huge book of pressure points for reflexology). He would adjust my spine, adjust my foot (huh?), have me hold a herbal supplement while he pushed down on my arm to test my body's reaction to being in contact with it (voodoo?), then he would have me touch my tongue to the roof of my mouth as he tapped his finger on my forehead. I thought this dude was cracked out, and I was dumb enough to participate. (I assumed this was being filmed as a new episode of the prank show "Punked.") BUT at the end of that first hour-long session, this guy had made more progress on my knee and how it felt than two years of doctors, physical therapists, MRI's, and x-rays had. SOLD!

Reflexology is based on the idea that your body has miles and miles of nerve fibers that move energy around your body. Reflexology works by manipulating the feet or hands or ears (where the nerves all dead end) with the intent of targeting certain organs to release energy blockages. Kind of like plucking different strings of a marionette to make the arms move versus another string to make the leg move.

For instance, massaging the arch of your foot corresponds to your spine. When I would have lower back pain or tightness after volleyball, I would massage and stimulate the proper area of my feet and hands, and literally, within an hour, the pain or tightness was dramatically reduced, if not gone altogether!

Here's how to try self-reflexology:

1. Take the underside of your foot and apply medium pressure with the tip of your thumb to different areas looking for a tender spot.
2. Look up on the chart what body part that corresponds to. (It's probably somewhere you are having a problem with.)
3. Apply medium pressure with the tip of your thumb to the spot for five to ten seconds while taking deep breaths. Release pressure then repeat. Do that for about a minute or two.
4. Give it time. It's not magic or voodoo. Repeat it a few times per hour. Drink water. Breathe the energy out. (Your body needs a way to remove blockage. Help it out.)

Use it for:

- Headaches – Big toe
- Back pain – along the foot arch
- Or 60 other areas

Intermittent Fasting

Fasting means no food. Intermittent fasting simply means eliminating food for a few hours, up to a few days, and following a regular pattern. Why would someone miss a perfectly good meal? Well, there is lots and lots of research that shows how your body reacts to short-term calorie restriction. The positive impacts include:

- Longer life expectancy
- Reduced blood glucose and insulin levels
- Increased fatty acid oxidation
- Muscle preservation
- Lower inflammation and lower blood pressure
- Leveled metabolism

Do I like IF (intermittent Fasting)?

YES! I think it's a great idea and a fantastic way to improve the above areas of the body and lower the doses of medications you're taking.

There is no one way to IF. It's part science, but it's really more art. And it's a symphonic harmony that we play with our individual bodies to find what makes us respond best. So now you have to choose:

- Skipped meal
- Condensed eating window
- Single 24-hour fast
- Alternating day fast
- 5:2 fasting

Many studies have shown impressive results in cholesterol and blood glucose levels in as little as two to three days of intermittent fasting. Fasting is FAST!

Is it a replacement for longer term fasting or the cleanses I recommend?

NO. I love that intermittent fasting requires less willpower than longer-term fasting/cleansing. I love that IF requires less of a lifestyle disruption than longer-term fasting/cleansing. I love that IF can create such awesome and measurable improvements in blood work and cholesterol. I highly recommend it as a regular activity to keep those vital blood indicators in check.

Then why not do more IF versus taking five to ten days to fast/cleanse? What does IF not do that we vitally need? Two things: 1) deep colon cleansing and 2) deeper cellular cleansing.

Simply fasting does not replace the colon cleansing power of the salt flush or other techniques to loosen and remove years of impacted fecal matter from your intestines. PERIOD.

That buildup of festering, bacteria-filled, toxic, leaking waste needs to be removed to give your body the fighting chance it needs to tip the healing scales in your favor.

With longer term fasting/cleansing, the combination of not eating (not adding new food that gets in the way of flushing the colon), nightly laxative teas (loosen the rock hard, impacted waste night after night after night), daily salt flushes (using sheer force to dislodge and loosen and wash away hardened waste day after day after day) is a benefit that IF can't achieve, in my opinion. (How was the Grand Canyon carved out of stone? Years and years of constant water flow.)

We are hacking into our bodies' systems to trigger body scavenging mode (autophagy – the body targets dysfunctional and damaged cells for breakdown in order to maintain energy levels). It takes around 48-72 hours to trigger that. That's what eats mutated cells, fat cells, cysts, crystals, garbage.

Sorry, no shortcut for that one!

13 Core Steps to Reset Your Body

1. 10-Day fasting detox
2. Drink 1/2 ounce of water per pound of your weight, daily
3. Eat three salads per day
4. No bread, no pasta.
5. Shoot for a 70% vegetable diet
6. No fast food
7. Sweat for fifteen minutes weekly
8. Work out four times per week
9. No drugs, no medications
10. Find the proper daily herbal supplements for you
11. Cleanse liver twice per year
12. 10-Day fasting detox annually and mid-year veggie cleanse
13. One cheat meal, once per week

10 Reasons Your Reset Isn't Working

1. Skipping or Omitting Steps

There are <u>13 Core Reset Steps</u>:

A) You have to do all the steps.
B) You have to do everything the step entails.

- You can't do everything, but continue to eat bread every day.
- You can't do the Veggie, or Juice, or Master Cleanse and skip the salt flush (or some other colon irrigating method as a replacement).
- You can't have a cheat DAY, it's a cheat meal.
- You can't do all these and not drink half your body weight in ounces of water daily.

It's like baking a cake. You need all the ingredients to make the cake right. If you leave the eggs out, how bad is that cake? Follow the recipe!

2. Inconsistency

-You can't try to average things out over a week. Every day millions of cells are dying and being created in your body. Every day counts. (Of course, wild life events will happen, but how often?)

-You can't eat one salad a day for a week then try to triple up on salads the next week.

-You can't go 18 months between annual cleanses.

-You can't workout one day a week

3. Too Much Processed Food

The chemicals and preservatives and antibiotics in most mass-produced food in America are constantly dumping more and more toxins into your body. Even if you cut back to a 70 percent vegetable diet and remove breads and pastas from your meals, if they are still laced with these energy sapping and toxic substances, your body is spending too much time and energy fighting them. Organic food will also deliver a far higher nutritional bang for your buck and feed your cells with "high-octane" fuel.

4. Not Working Out

You can't skip this step unless you are ok with slower results. Have people been able to hit their Reset goals without working out? YES. Does it take longer? YES

Keep in mind that working out four days a week can look like lots of things. It does NOT mean that you have to be throwing weights around in a gym, running marathons, or jellifying your body with CrossFit workouts (BUT if you are bad-ass enough to do those things, you'll see and feel the difference). Maybe you'll jump rope, hula-hoop, jog, or use a DVD home workout, BUT the key is to push yourself and shock and surprise your body. If you already work out, then get a trainer. If you hit the gym hard, then pick up a sport. Keep your body from being able to fire on auto mode and get bored with your workout and thus gain no challenge from the workout.

5. You Need More Frequent Cleansing

Once a year of a fasting cleanse and a mid-year Veggie Cleanse and the occasional 1-Day Reset will be enough for many of you to hit your health goal and maintain it for the rest of your life. But guess what? Your name isn't "many of you," so you may need to do more to get more. You may be old and have decades of toxins or fat or deeper seeded illnesses. You may be trying to lose 100 or more pounds of fat. You may just have a stubborn body. There could be a lot of reasons. It really doesn't matter why. You just need more!

If you're trying to lose 100 pounds or more of fat, you can perform the Master/Juice Cleanses every 30 days (give your body a 30-day rest period in between to give it time to repair and build itself up to prepare for the next round).

You may need to do 1-Day Resets more often to undo damage from lacking discipline with your eating habits. You can do the 1-Day Reset with no limitations for as long as you like (days in a row, weeks in a row). It's great for your body. NOTE: If you decide to do it for weeks at a time, you don't need to do two daily salt flushes. One a day is fine. And be sure to add cultured foods and probiotics to your diet to replenish the good bacteria being flushed away.

Remember, the longer each cleanse, the deeper it repairs. So a ten-day cleanse will be FAR more beneficial than two five-day cleanses with rest in between. Maybe you need to work your way up from a five-day cleanse to ten-day cleanses. Think of it this way:

Imagine your cleanse process as a group of lumberjacks chopping trees deep into a fast-growing forest. On day one, they hack in ten feet. Then they rest at night. On day two they start already at ten feet in, and they hack in ten feet more. Now they are twenty feet in. So every day they are able to start where they left off the night before. BUT if they take a day off, ten feet will grow back. So as long as those little lumberjacks keep working every day, they'll go deeper and deeper.

6. Medications

I've seen situations where the drugs or medications someone was taking were severely slowing down their Reset. NOTE: I'm not saying to go cold turkey and end your medications. That's between you and your doctor. Use your common sense, please. At the same time, take responsibility for your life and success. Pay attention to your body. Only you can feel what you're feeling.

Some medications cause many side effects and they wreak havoc on your body's systems. Sometimes the dosage can be so high the residual toxic load is just too much for your body to remove every day. Sometimes people have allergies or exaggerated reactions to a particular medication. The drug still does what it's prescribed for, but it can also cause an inflammatory reaction that has its own issues.

7. Allergies

There are thousands of stories of people with a daily routine or a family tradition – a thing they drink (a tea or juice) or eat (a snack or a type of vegetable) – that they have had an allergic reaction to all their life and had no idea. A man has had lifelong sneezing. Not terrible, but a big annoyance. Every morning, since childhood, he has his mom's recipe tea. One time he leaves town for a week, has no tea. Amazingly enough, no sneezing! CURED. Then he returns home, goes back to his tea. SNEEZING again. It took him 30 years, but he figured it out.

You may have some sort of food allergy that is slowing or altogether stopping your body from making further progress to reach your goal. A particular food might be making you constipated, turning into fat easily, causing skin issues, causing inflammation (breathing issues, joint pain, etc.) and causing water retention. Anything.

You may need to start removing certain foods from your diet, one at a time, and keeping a food journal to note your body's reaction (start with the foods that you have eaten the longest). A great time to do this is when you are coming off of a fast (Juice/Master Cleanse). Slowly start adding foods back into your diet, four days at a time, and note how they affect you. Patience is key here.

8. Not Using Herbal Supplementation

More often than not, people will skip Core Step # 10 – Find The Right Herbal Supplements for You. It's the "for you" part that is most important. After a lifetime of damage and toxins targeted at your weak spot, more often than not, it will need a boost and a leg up to function normally again. Medicinal herbs are the boost, the hack, the way to naturally target your weak spot for special attention. In my case, with my joints being my weak spot (bad ankles, bad knees, bad shoulders), after a lot of experimentation, I found what gives me the boost I need – daily fish oil (lubes my joints), daily turmeric (anti-inflammatory) along with tons of daily water and a mostly vegetable diet. They were the punch that I needed, and still need to this day, to maintain my equilibrium. But I had to play around with different fish oils (liquid vs. capsule, cod liver vs Udo's oil, etc.).

Yours might be a sluggish bowel and constipation issues, so aloe vera oil taken orally might be a supplement you need. Maybe you have wild digestive issues so probiotic supplements would help you. Or you seem to get colds a lot. Daily garlic intake or ginger teas might be your herbs of choice. Maybe you're dealing with prostate issues. Saw palmetto could help you. Migraines, low energy, poor eyesight, acne, yeast infections, insulin deficiencies, erectile dysfunction, low sex drive, and thousands more issues can be addressed with the proper herbal supplementation once your body has Reset enough for your systems to be able to do what they were made to do.

9. Deep-Seated Disease

Here is a sad fact. There are those that have had a disease for so long and their lifestyle has hammered it deeper and deeper into their body's organs, that it reaches the point where the detoxification of the illness causes such violent and prolonged pain and discomfort, they don't have the time or stamina to endure it. That, my friends, is what doctors, drugs, and medications were created for. And they are stellar at doing the job. Using standard doctors, drugs, and medications is not bad. But the daily reliance on them is. Ask any doctor: they don't want you having to come see them for the rest of your life. They want to you heal and get better and not have to be on the cocktail of meds that you currently are on.

If you are like me and do everything in your power to not have to visit a doctor or take a drug or medication BUT in your case you have a deep-rooted disease or illness that you haven't been able to get under control, don't be closed off to temporary medical intervention. TEMPORARILY, to balance the scales long enough for your natural efforts to win out. Think about it, we are exposed to very unnatural toxins and man-made chemicals and high concentrations of germs and odd organisms that our bodies have not had a chance to adapt to over the years. So why not fight fire with fire? Not every day for the rest of your life, but if you have had a lifelong Candida yeast over growth throughout your body, why not combine your natural Candida protocol with a couple of weeks of Diflucan or another medical antifungal? If you have lifelong issues with bladder or other bacterial infections, don't be too proud to use antibiotics for a few weeks – just long enough for your natural efforts to win over (and be diligent in replacing any beneficial bacteria when you have completed the antibiotics).

Do I recommend surgery? NO. NEVER. Once we open up the body, tinker around removing things, cutting organs, removing bones, fusing bones, etc. it complicates things that much more for your body's healing systems. (Obviously, if you are in an accident, get all the emergency surgeries needed to save your life.) Chronic diseases and illnesses might not be easy to treat and correct without surgery in lots of cases, but I never said it was easy. But it's worth it!

10. Stress and Mental State

In America, we tend to downplay the physical impacts of stress and mindset. THEY ARE REAL! And they manifest in physical ailments just as easily as bacteria and viruses. Believe it.

Your body is a very simple machine. When your brain needs to send signals through your nervous systems, many times it uses chemicals to get the message across. Stress produces chemicals called hormones – cortisol and epinephrine. The chemicals aren't bad (we're not talking about Clorox bleach) but just like any other chemical, it is a toxin (your body can't digest or assimilate it). But as long as we flush the chemicals out as fast as stress produces them, they don't build up and cause harm. Imagine you're in a tiny rowboat. As you get stressed, water leaks into your boat through a little hole in the bottom. But as long as you stick to a Reset lifestyle that removes those chemicals, you are able to bail out the water in your tiny boat before it fills up. BUT if that hole gets larger (lots of constant stress) and you aren't bailing fast enough (not removing the chemical hormones fast enough), it's simple logic that your boat will fill (starting with your weak spots) and eventually you will sink. Simple as that!

REDUCE YOUR STRESS.

The same thing occurs with a negative mental attitude. As hocus pocus as it sounds, holding on to a pessimistic outlook on life, focusing on what's wrong instead of focusing on what's right, always seeing the glass as half empty, being distrustful of others with no provocation – these things absolutely will hold you back and prevent you from making the health progress you deserve. Have you ever had a headache for a while then forgotten about it? Then someone asks you, "How's your headache?" All of a sudden, you start to feel it again? Crazy, huh? If you focus your energy on a thing, you will tend to get that thing.

CHANGE YOUR THOUGHTS, CHANGE YOUR HEALTH.

GOOD NEWS: There will come a point where your body reaches an equilibrium, and you won't need to be as strict with your 13 Steps. For me it happened after about four years. From day one I felt and saw benefits (from my first cleanse, to stopping fast food, to drinking water, etc.) I could track and see it was working regularly, but after four years, I could eat breads and pasta with less bloating. When I hit that equilibrium, I could skip a few salads before I felt it in my joints. After equilibrium, I no longer CRAVED processed foods or sweets so I didn't need to use willpower. They just weren't on my radar any longer!

That equilibrium will happen for you. You may be one of the lucky ones, and one cleanse Resets your body. Or it could take you years (with tons of noticeable, trackable life improvements along the way). But when it happens, you can cheat more, slack more, be free more. But YOU. MUST. EARN. IT.

I did. And you will too. BE WELL.

SELECTED BLOG POSTS

I've been back in America for two weeks and I'm pissed!

I'm pissed because I've been living in places that are NOT plagued with obesity and cancer and heart disease and diabetes.

I'm pissed because I've been living in places where the government is outlawing dangerous substances and, oddly, PROTECTING the citizens' interests over the profit of corporations.

Are these people more worthy than us?
Have these people suffered more than us?
Do these people deserve better than us?
Do they have better doctors?
Do they have more money?
Are they special?

I lived in Stockholm, Sweden, for four months and traveled to Denmark, The Netherlands, Norway, Turkey, Greece, and the Czech Republic over the past year. Prior to that, I have been able to visit Brazil, Colombia, Australia, Canada, and Mexico. What have I witnessed relating to health on my travels?

1. The countries with the healthiest populations (in my opinion) have very little overweight citizens. (I'm not talking about people running around with six-pack abs or gym rats. I'm talking about regularly built people with no excess fat on their bodies and no outwardly visible signs of extraordinarily poor health.)

2. Just like us, they eat what is around them and most available. They are not running around desperately seeking low calorie, "healthy" super foods. They eat out of convenience, too.

3. They are gym fanatics any more than your average big-city American. "But they walk so much more, Terry!" Anyone live in New York City? Or Chicago? That's how much they walk too.

What gives? What's the deal??

More than 3,000 food additives – preservatives, flavorings, colors, and other ingredients – are added to US foods. About 150 of those chemicals are banned in many of the countries that I've visited with the healthiest populations, including genetically modified foods.
http://articles.mercola.com/sites/articles/archive/2013/02/27/us-food-products.aspx

And furthermore, the Food Babe published a spectacular article (http://foodbabe.com/tag/ingredients-banned-in-other-countries/) on how many US food corporations reformulate foreign versions of the same foods we eat here, "leaving out almost all of the questionable ingredients in the non-US versions."

The fact of the matter is, if you feed humans chemicals, it makes them fatter and sicker. PERIOD.

"But what about all the testing and studies that don't prove that conclusively?"

I imagine some old European official that had ancestral roots in his country for a thousand years being asked to approve the torrent of chemical additives for his country. He looks at the corporate representative and says, "You're asking me to allow you to experiment on my family's traditions and food supply in exchange for a very large sum of money. I would like you to leave my office and my country and never return. I have to look these people in the eye."

But for some reason we said OK to the chemical storm. To make for better crop yields. To make for prettier fruits and vegetables. To make for livestock that can survive through their disease-ridden upbringing. To make for longer shelf life at the grocery store. To make for a better marketing angle to beat out the competition. **How's that little experiment been working out for the past 30 years?**

People should NOT have to be busting their ass at the gym seven days a week just to maintain!

Two of every three Americans are overweight. (Look to your left, now look to your right. Two of you are, on average, about 32lbs over weight)

One out of every three Americans is obese. That means 78 MILLION Americans are 61 pounds or more overweight. Or 100lbs overweight. Or 200lbs overweight.

THAT'S UNACCEPTABLE.

"European portion sizes are so much smaller than American portions"

Well of course they are! Think of it this way. You have a:
Scooter (it takes scooter fuel -weak)

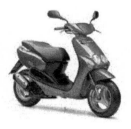

Automobile (it takes automobile fuel – stronger)

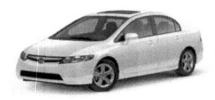

Jet Plane (it takes jet fuel – strongest)

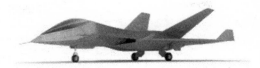

You are the jet plane. But you're being given scooter fuel. You need more fuel. Larger portions (and calorie) needs. PERIOD.

We have it in our grasp to fix it. It's not magic.

It breaks my heart to go to the gym and see so many hardworking people slaving to lose 50, 100, 150 pounds. I honor them. I admire their tenacity. What I see when I look at them are soldiers on the battlefield. But what these soldiers don't know is that their commander sent them into battle armed with rifles shooting blanks. But that isn't stopping them from fighting for what they believe. They are close enough to the enemy now that they are using their rifles to club their foe. They are fighting with their fists, tooth and nail. These stubborn, unstoppable soldiers are fighting their uphill battle in spite of the handicap given them by their superiors. That's courage. That's bravery. Those are my kind of people.

IT DOES NOT HAVE TO BE THIS HARD.

"But corporations will lose too much money"

Listen. We use millions to subsidize crap food, crap chemicals, and counterproductive farming. We have the money. We can even entertain the idea of subsidizing these large companies for a couple of years for them to retool and remove the chemicals and genetic modification.

THEY CAN ADAPT OR DIE.

"But it will take forever to change the system"

BULL CRAP! If we got wind that there was a major poisoning of a certain food coming out of a factory and it was causing deaths, we would shut that factory down – OVERNIGHT – and remove any suspected tainted food from shelves – OVERNIGHT.

NEWSFLASH! There IS poison making it into our food supply and it IS causing deaths. They just aren't happening right away. We are not a weak, frail species, we humans. It's taken YEARS for kids to come down with childhood-onset diabetes. It's taken years for teens to graduate to the obesity category.

The American 20

Start asking around, and you'll hear tale after tale of Americans that visited certain countries, maintained their lifestyle and eating habits, and lost significant amounts of weight. Or even had lifelong diseases fade away. ASK!

You'll also hear tales of foreigners that visited America only to have the American 20 hit them square in the gut, those 20 pounds you gain just by living off the most prevalent food around you.

The answer is education and teaching people what to eat.

Ridiculous waste of time and resources.

"Dear American citizens, you have all been given access to some very complicated and varying, non-exact information that, if you choose to ignore it (as we all know 80 percent of people pay zero attention to optional educational resources), will result in your being bombarded with cheaper, more available, sweeter food options that you already are biologically addicted to. Soon your heart disease, cancer, obesity, and diabetes rates will skyrocket and we will spend billions in health care to manage those. If only you had read the book we gave you. Good luck" – Uncle Sam

Why not just give a toddler a full-color schematic of street traffic patterns and leave him on the side of a busy intersection? "Good luck, tiger; be sure you read that before you chase this ball I'm throwing out there."

It should be the responsibility of our elected government to create an environment that doesn't require constant second-guessing and high-level nutrition education on the predominant food choices in a nation. We have enough life drama to contend with – primary education, higher education, employment, family building, and pursuit of happiness – that we don't need to be playing food roulette three times a day for the sake of corporate irresponsibility and laziness.

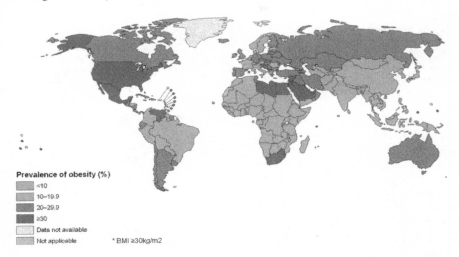

Prevalence of obesity (%)
- <10
- 10–19.9
- 20–29.9
- ≥30
- Data not available
- Not applicable   * BMI ≥30kg/m2

It worked with cigarettes: Make the bad stuff harder to get and tax the hell out of it!

I believe in freedom of the market and freedom of choice. If someone wants to find re-released Twinkies…let 'em. If someone needs a high-fructose corn syrup fix, let them have it. But make it a more expensive product.

Give subsidies to products with no chemical additives.

Set age restrictions on products that contain too many of the more questionable chemical additives.

How will I know that we've made it? When I'm walking past a corner store and I overhear a kid asking an adult, "Hey, mister, can I give you $10 and you buy me a bag of Honey BBQ Cheetos Puffs?"

I'm pissed that my father has to sit in a hospital and fight for his health when all he did wrong is eat food.

I'm pissed that my mother has to fight so hard to silence the temptation song of a quart of ice cream.

I'm pissed that my grandmother is fighting Alzheimer's but her symptoms improve when I'm there to correct her diet.

I'm pissed that my best friend's mother died because of cancer.

I'm pissed that my friend had heart surgery in his 30s.

I'm pissed that my friend had to fight to survive breast cancer in her 30s.

Can you tell that I'm pissed?

Do you disagree? Great. Do you REALLY DISAGREE? Even better! Email me. Make some noise. The more attention the better!

Do you agree with what I'm saying? Does it FEEL right in your gut? Then:

1. Start buying organic when you can
2. Avoid tap water with chlorine and fluoride
3. Join my mailing list
4. Visit the Food Policy site www.foodpolicyaction.org (contact your legislators, etc.)
5. Share this information with five people

Get off the fence and do something! We have enough people sitting around nodding their heads and agreeing.

I need some more soldiers. They may have given us rifles shooting blanks, but with the right army, we can win this battle. Up close. We see the whites of their eyes. We feel the heat of their breath. Come with me.

With passion and numbers, a revolution can be born.

Today

I **could go outside today!** The weather is breathtaking. The skies are clear. I see a gentle breeze in the trees. But this nagging pain in my knee. Ugh. I don't want to aggravate it today. What if it throws off my getting to and from work? **No outside today.**

I could hit the gym today! Bang out a few sets on the rack machine. Get the old blood flowing! Knock off the cobwebs and get back into my old routine of working out three or four days a week. It's sometimes a drudgery to get there, but the rush I feel afterwards, the surge of power, the feeling of accomplishment that makes it all worth it! But I have ZERO energy and even less time. Ugh. I'm doing enough just to make it through these long days at work lately. And when would I even be able to go? If only I had more hours in my day. **No gym today. Maybe next week.**

I could lay out in the sun today! It's so rare for the stars to align and the best weather to fall on my day off. I feel like this is a day that songs are written about. Not too hot, not too cold. I have nothing else going on. I'm looking a bit pale, and I'm not part vampire. That vitamin D is just what I need. But I'm not looking like the high school prom queen I used to be. Ugh. I know there is more to me than how I think I look, and I couldn't care less what other people think about how I look in a bathing suit but why even waste the time? My bikini is out of date. I'm not in the mood to go try on new ones and spend money. And everyone is lying around judging one another when you walk by:

"Her boobs are too this," "Her butt is too that," "That bathing suit is too much/ too little."' I'm not a piece of meat. **No lying out today.**

I could go play some ball today! Sitting here at this traffic light watching these guys go at it. Ahh. I had my signature move that nobody could stop. I'd get the call from the boys and skip work or show up late to my next obligation. I just lost track of time out there. Game after game. Then I'd come back the next day and do it all over again. I should have been discovered! But the last few times, I kept throwing my back out. And all the other minor injuries here and there just kept taking longer and longer to heal. Messed up my work schedule too. **Nah, no ball today.**

I could take an exciting vacation to a foreign country and walk around the endless historical sites of ages ago! Many of the cities and sites of those lands were built long before cars and freeways. I could truly take in the culture and my ancestry and be hands on. Treading the cobblestone roads, climbing to the summit of the royal monuments, following in the footsteps of the explorers that blazed trails in this wilderness. My own adventure! But my daily medication needs and the fact that I'm out of breath simply hiking these damn stairs and walking down my long driveway to check mail make that sound less like a vacation and more like servitude. **No hiking vacations today.**

Just because you can't do it today, doesn't mean that that you can't do it tomorrow.

Start Resetting your body.

Grow younger as you age.

You owe it to yourself...BE WELL.

Ladies – Get larger, fuller breasts (1-2 cups sizes), naturally!

I get that breasts and breast size can have a major effect on some women's self-confidence, but not all women. It's not like women are just walking bosom displays, but I know it is a pretty prominent display of sexuality.

Eating a nutrient-dense and chemical-free diet during puberty has radical effects on how the adult ends up.

Does that mean that we have to live with the mistake of our early lifestyle choices forever? NOPE.

So let's say, for whatever your personal reason, you want larger, fuller, natural breasts. Here's how.

Question - When do women's breasts grow the most?

Answer – Puberty.

Essentially, to get your breasts to grow again, we need to re-create the same hormonal conditions that were present when you were in puberty. We do this by manipulating the hormones inside your body to make your breasts "think" that it's time to grow again. Period!

Then we maintain a high-nutrient diet delivering all the building blocks that your body needs to accomplish the task at hand.

Estrogen is the main hormone that determines the size of your breasts. Not only does it make your breasts bigger and more rounded, it affects other parts of your body too.

Getting the estrogen levels right inside your body is the first step to getting bigger breasts. However, it's not as simple as increasing the estrogen levels inside your body as many women think. The timing, the combination of the correct hormones, ensuring the body delivers the right hormones to the right places – these are the trickier parts.

Simple overview:

- Iodine supplementing
- Herbal supplementing starting first day of period
- One capsule of each of these herbs, three times per day: red clover, fenugreek and saw palmetto
- Last day of period, stop the herbs (continue with iodine)
- Three months on herbs, one month off herbs
- By four months, you should gain a cup size
- Most women reach their goal by six months

Iodine Supplementing:

Americans are in the middle of an iodine deficiency epidemic right now.

Why?

- In the 1920s, the government implemented iodized salt to address the epidemic. It worked! BUT now we don't eat as much iodized salt
- Fluoride, chlorine, and bromine in our food and water supply block the body's absorption of iodine

Iodine is critical for a properly functioning thyroid. The thyroid controls the body's production of hormones. Those hormones control how much testosterone is produced in men.

It does not take much and it does not take long to see some pretty drastic changes once you start iodine supplementing!

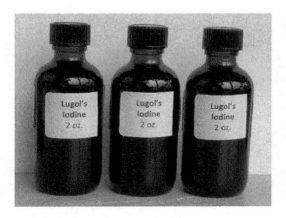

I recommend:

- Lugol's Solution
- It's iodine in a solution of potassium iodide
- Buy it online or at a health store
- It will be anywhere from 2%-5% in strength (get whatever you can. Don't stress)
- It could take about a year to correct a deficiency so you may start with 1-2 drops in water and then gradually work your way up to 6-8 drops, twice daily. Then after a year, come back down to a maintenance dose of 1-2 drops in water, daily.

Important! If you go too fast, you may experience some detox reactions:

- sore throat
- headache
- feeling depressed
- skin eruptions

In that case, simply lower your dose by a drop or two until they pass.

- Eat plenty of sea salt daily

That's it. To really accelerate things you can incorporate progesterone cream as well as breast massaging.

Jenny Bolton sells a FAR more comprehensive and resourceful product filled with more suggestions. (I make no profit from any sales) For more information visit: http://boostyourbust.com/

What to expect:

- Growth pain (remember puberty?)
- Breast swelling
- Mood swings (it comes with the territory)
- Tiredness (don't fight it)
- Irregular periods

Big note: these work best and most reliably if you have a clean, healthy diet (read my six rules for eating naturally and clean) and ESPECIALLY if you incorporate cleansing once or twice per year to help remove the backlog of decades of toxic build up is in your body and organs.

Guys: Get Bigger Cohones, More Testosterone, and More Sex Drive

First, I found research like this:

"You are half the man your grandfather was! This generation's testosterone levels are half what they were in the 1950s and dropping by one percent each year."

Then I read a study about a little experiment where two baby calves were raised, one on raw milk, the other on pasteurized milk, and the resulting differences were listed and compared with photos.

http://thebovine.wordpress.com/2010/06/04/the-tale-of-two-calves-one-calf-got-raw-milk-the-other-pasteurized/

After five months:

Calf #1 (Raw milk)

Not only was he twice as big, his hair was shinier, he was far more alert, his liver (after slaughter) had a healthier color, his kidney (after slaughter) had a healthier color and a firmer consistency, his belly (after slaughter) was filled with better, more consistent contents that did not stink like the other calf.

BUT! The most striking difference for me was the testes. HOLY COW! (Get it?)

The pasteurized cow's testes were shriveled up, small, tight, and snug to his body.

But the raw milk calf's (I call him Mandingo), that dude's testes were larger, healthy looking, full, and ready for action. I'm not a lady cow, but if I were, I imagine I'd be aroused!

What gives?

Is this about milk? NO.

This is about nutrition and how it affects Mother Nature's master plan of having the strong survive.

Pasteurized milk (the stuff most humans drink) is heated to 150 degrees for 30 minutes to kill potential harmful bacteria in it. BUT it also destroys much of the nutritional benefits of the live contents of the milk.

(All this REQUIRED pasteurization of our milk is really a byproduct of corporate megafarm neglect and non-localization of the milk, but I'll write about that another time.)

Not enough nutrients in your food during puberty (just like calf #2) will force your body to make do with what it receives.

After seeing this, I wondered, what if I purposely raised my own testosterone levels? What would happen to me?

Ready to feel 21-years-old in the sack again? GO!

1. Iodine Supplementing

Americans are in the middle of an iodine deficiency epidemic right now.

Why?

- In the 1920s, the government implemented iodized salt to address the epidemic. It worked! BUT now we don't eat as much iodized salt.
- Fluoride, chlorine, and bromine in our food and water supply, block the body's absorption of iodine.

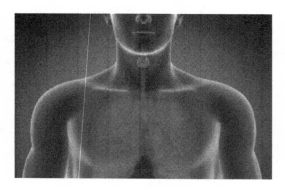

Iodine is critical for a properly functioning thyroid. The thyroid controls the body's production of hormones. Those hormones control how much testosterone men produce.

It does not take much and it does not take long to see some pretty drastic changes once you start iodine supplementing!

I recommend:

Lugol's Solution

- It's iodine in a solution of potassium iodide
- Buy it online or at a health store
- It will be anywhere from 2%-5% in strength (get whatever you can. Don't stress.)
- It could take about a year to correct a deficiency so you may start with 1-2 drops in water and then gradually work your way up to 6-8 drops, twice daily. Then after a year, come back down to a maintenance dose of 1-2 drops in water, daily.

Important! If you go too fast, you may experience some detox reactions:

- sore throat
- headache
- feeling depressed
- skin eruptions

In that case, simply lower your dose by a drop or two until they pass.

- Eat plenty of sea salt daily

2. Eat more healthy fats. Men turn fat into testosterone.

GOOD FATS:

- Avocado
- Coconut oil
- Nuts and seeds (almonds, sunflower seeds, etc.)
- Grass-fed cow butter

3. Cold Showers

It's simple. They've tested testosterone levels before the cold shower and after it. The levels were higher. DO IT!

- No hot water
- Do it every day
- As long or as quick as you like
- MAN UP! Cold water won't kill you bro

4. No masturbation, no porn

Ready? Stimulating your caveman brain with 100 different naked writhing women each night ain't natural! Study after study shows that it desensitizes the male brain and thus requiring MORE stimulation to keep him (and Mr. Happy) happy.

After three to four weeks, if the wind as much blows, you'll be ready to go into battle. And your testosterone levels increase more when you're not wasting precious soldiers on two-dimensional erotica.

Matt Cook sells a fantastic product in hyperboosting testosterone. For more details, more resources (I receive no profits from any sales), visit:

http://www.datingskillsreview.com/testosterone-rewind-the-testosterone-liftoff-formula/

Big note: these work best and most reliably if you have a clean, healthy diet (read my six rules for eating naturally and clean) and ESPECIALLY if you incorporate cleansing once or twice per year to help remove whatever backlog of decades of crazy toxic buildup is in your body and organs.

Eating a nutrient-dense and chemical-free diet during puberty has radical effects on how the adult ends up.

Does that mean that we have to live with the mistake of our early lifestyle choices forever? NOPE.

Speaking & Employee Wellness Program

Unless you are retired, I'm willing to wager a large sum of money that one of these applies to you: a) you work at a company or b) you own or run a company. Statistically speaking, the employees at said company are 30 pounds overweight, they take 2-4 medications daily, they are having surgeries, they have a hard time waking in the mornings, they want to fall asleep at 2 p.m. every day, they head home exhausted, eat fast food for dinner, watch TV, and then crash to do it over the next day. They deserve better. They are frustrated, they want to change, but they don't know how.

What does that do?

Sick employees, employees in pain, and unhappy employees make it EXCEEDINGLY difficult for your company to succeed at whatever vision it is striving for. All that leads to less productivity, more paid time off, less engagement in the work place, less energy to bring your company's vision to life. What would a 1% increase in productivity mean to your financial bottom line?

If you would like to learn more about how I help employees say, "My employer actually cares about my welfare!" and how that leads to lowered monthly premiums, less paid time off, a more energetic work force, a more positive work force, far better engaged employee bonding and support, and less cash wellness incentives.

Contact my team directly at support@TerryGivens.com or online at www.TerryGivens.com.

Pay It Forward

Thank you for buying Reset Your Body, the handbook to help you naturally grow younger as you age! I know that you work hard for the money you spend, and that when you spend it, you trust you will receive value. I promise that you will find value in each page of this book, value enough that it has changed the lives of hundreds. So I ask you one simple thing – if you find value in these pages, please take a few moments to pay it forward by leaving me a brief review so that others can find value as you have. Thank you and BE WELL.

Join Us!

Now that you know what to do, come join us so that you don't have to do it alone! Join my online Reset Support Group; it's free! Join thousands of folks that want to grow younger as they age. Get questions answered, interact with others like you, cheer each other on, and be held accountable. The key to success is action and consistency, let's do it together!

www.ResetYourBody.com/SupportGroup

About the Author

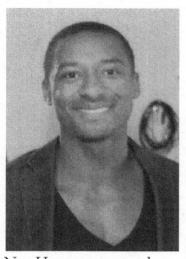

"I'm just a normal guy trying to help people."

Terry lives in Pacific Beach, California and is an admitted beach addict. Beach volleyball, travelling abroad often, and enjoying live music tops his "Heaven on Earth" list.

He was not a health nut born to hippy parents who raised him on a mountainside, teaching him to respect nature and the cycle of life. No. He was a normal guy from the Midwest, raised to eat meat and potatoes and not make a big deal out of it. By high school, the standard American diet had taken its toll on him by ravaging his hip joints. In college, he began having problems with his ankles. He had shoulder injuries and a surgery in his twenties, and his knees were ineffective for sports by just his early 30s. Terry rationalized his suffering with the "I'm just getting old" mantra...BULL CRAP!

After a chance exposure to the right information and the right people, he began to rebuild, restore, and reset his body. Now a certified nutritionist, he reveals seven years of research, experimentation, and expert interviews that led to a 41-year-old Terry looking and feeling younger, stronger, and more energetic than he did at when he was 25.

Summed up into 8 Reset Challenges, it's a proven system that's doable for real people with real lives. It's believable, and it's helping thousands to become younger as they age. This could be the very thing you've been waiting for.

Made in the USA
Middletown, DE
17 September 2016